I0417206

THE BEAUTY BOOKS

Oil Belly, Flat Belly

———————

Sonja Y. Larsen

Oil Belly, Flat Belly (The Beauty Books, Book 2)
Copyright © 2015 by Blue Sun Media

All rights reserved. No part of this book may be reproduced or transmitted in any form or by any means without written permission from the author.

ISBN 978-1512113419

Printed in USA

Disclaimer

It is an absolute condition of sale of this book that you consult with your doctor or health care practitioner before practicing any of the methods described in this book. This book is for educational purposes only and is not intended to treat, cure or prevent any condition or disease. The author shall not be held responsible or liable for any loss or damage from any suggestion or information contained in this book.

Why You Need To Read This Book

Alas, there's hope without doing a thousand abdominal crunches per day. Like we'd ever do a thousand anyway. Heck, one hundred isn't even happening for many of us. We know we should, but we don't because it doesn't seem to even make a big difference in the battle of the bulge anyway.

But we do see them off yonder. The ones with bellies nice enough to wear just a sports bra and shorts to the gym...the ones that don't have to suck it in for a proposed group Facebook picture...the ones that fit into things without a big pot belly hanging over.

It seems like no matter what we do, there it is. Forget the six-pack; some of us are just trying not to look 4-6 months pregnant. Are guys even looking for six-pack women? It seems like flatness with a slight curvature is sexy enough. Even if you wanted to get to six-packdom, you would need to remove fat first, then build abdominal muscles afterward. It doesn't simply turn straight from fat to muscle all in one go. That is probably why you are struggling to make great abs at the gym. It won't work because abs are made in the kitchen.

This means that once you rid of unwanted belly fat at home, you can then begin building a six pack at the gym. The six-pack is optional, of course. This book begins at the beginning—the part where you flush fat down the toilet and button your jeans without heaving and panting. It does not begin with crunches, ab wheel rollouts, sit-ups, or flutter kicks.

How do we accomplish this? Sit back, relax, and enjoy this flat belly book. You're about to find out how to lose fat with natural, edible oils. You'll slather them on your body, you'll eat them, and you'll drink them.

No really, sit back and relax. Read this book and you'll discover a safe and effective way to flatten your belly without crunches or sit-ups. You will lose fat in a natural, healthy way—no liposuction, no tummy-tuck, no gastric bypass surgery. You will literally be laying around without lifting a finger while you anoint your belly with detoxifying, healing oils. You will be putting oils like castor oil, olive oil, and coconut oil to work for you. It won't be hard, but it will take some effort to gather and prepare ingredients. Once you begin using oils for your belly, your belly will get busy moving and working for a healthier you. It is about being healthy, right? The belly fat loss is just a by-product of the healthier you. Not only can you get rid of the bulge, but you can rid your belly of conditions like:

- o Fibroids
- o Ovarian Cysts
- o Adhesions
- o Internal Scars
- o Gas
- o Bloating
- o Indigestion
- o IBS

If you still want to do crunches later, then by all means go for it!

Table of Contents

Introduction

In year 2000 I was the heaviest I had ever been, weighing in at 210 pounds. My feet ached and I had to buy bigger, roomier clothing all the time. I even fell a couple times, because my poor little ankles could not balance all the weight I was packing on. I am not big-boned. There was just no excuse for how heavy I was. One day I got sick and tired of being too heavy.

In December 2000, I started going to the gym every day, joining fun aerobic classes, and watching portion size. I gradually took off 45 pounds over the next 3 years, landing at 165. I hung out at around 165 for several years, not reaching my goal of 145.

I'm 5'5", so 165 is not super fat, but it sure as heck isn't optimum either. I really wasn't happy with the way I looked, even though I religiously worked out and ate healthy. I could not seem to shake that last 20 pounds. I was on a five-year plateau.

The worst part was my belly. It was huge. What was in there? It was a mystery to me. I ate lots of green organic foods, did colon cleanses, and tried to do lots of abs. But I still had this big belly that looked like I was downing a case of beer every night.

What I discovered was that I had inflammation, fat, mucous, and Candida trapped in my belly. No matter how many kale smoothies I pushed through my system, no matter how often I purchased and used cleansing formulas, and no matter how many crunches I did, the gunk did not go away. The food came and left, but the mucous and Candida clung to my intestinal tract and uterus and stayed there. How do I know? Because I later flushed it all down the toilet.

Fast forward to the year 2014, and my belly is flat, my skin is glowing, and my energy is through the roof. You may have read my book about oil pulling, called "Oil Pulling (The Beauty Books, Book 1)". I share my personal success story, along with some how-to information, and guidance. Oil pulling was just the beginning of my oil journey. Later I found that using oils to cleanse and anoint my body was one of the best beauty secrets I could have ever discovered. I've been living with oils ever since.

What did I do? I began using oils to cleanse and discard fat from my body. And it worked. I used fat to get rid of fat. I'm not a scientist by any stretch of the imagination, but I like to focus on one simple chemistry mantra that says, "Like dissolves like."

One day I commented to my husband that I like to keep it simple and minimize when it comes to beauty products, "...cause I'm low-maintenance."

I got a blank stare. So I followed it up with, "Don't you think I'm low-maintenance, Honey?"

"No, Cutie...there's not a lot of oils and things here," he replied. Good answer.

If you came to our apartment, you would find oils on the sofa side table, in the refrigerator, in the cabinet above the stove, and in the bathroom. You would even find a set of oils sitting next to my head when I sleep at night.

I guess all women like to imagine they're low-maintenance, and just naturally beautiful. But what I mean is that I like a minimalistic natural beauty regimen—one that leaves out all the chemicals. And I like to do it myself. I decide what goes in my body, and on my body. Instead of buying a product containing almond oil, I buy the almond oil. I run from products that claim they will soften my skin, yet contain long words I cannot pronounce.

At the time I am writing this book, I am 42. Yet I look and feel younger and younger every year. Someone told me just yesterday that I look 24, not 42.

Think of me as the Tin Man in the Wizard of Oz who was stiff and rusty until Dorothy sprayed some lube on him. Then all of a sudden he was shaking and dancing. Fat is sliding off my body, all my joints move easily, and my skin has never looked better.

I have been using oils to cleanse and dispel yucky things from my body for a number of years. I would like to share some things that I have learned along the way.

Chapter One

Abs Are Made in the Kitchen

"Let food be thy medicine, and medicine be thy food."—
Hippocrates

Belly fat has everything to do with what you put in your
mouth. Indeed, exercise and sweating is a vital component to
good health. You need to sweat regularly to stay young,
healthy, and beautiful. However, a workout at the gym is not a
free ticket to consume whatever you want. In order to lose belly
fat, you must place the majority of effort into your daily
nutrition plan. Your flat belly will probably never come if you:
A. Starve yourself and then binge later, B. Pig out at happy
hour as a reward for working out, or C. Eat processed food
every day.

The Hoarding of Fat

We are modern beings living in the same bodies as those
who lived before us. Only now, we consume processed food-like
substances, and we spin wheels to consume them faster.

When your body senses a shortage of food, it begins
hoarding fat. This is the way we function. Humans survived
and thrived this way before they could make a pit stop at the
neighborhood market. We used to have to hunt or gather our
meals. Now we just pass by the fast food drive-thru lane on the
way home.

It was feast or famine for our ancestors, and their bodies
adapted ways of coping through times of famine. Perhaps a
draught occurred, or a hunter returned with no meat. Maybe

the ground was still frozen from winter, and food was hard to come by.

Your body responds to starvation by hoarding fat. It's your body's way of shutting down energy-burning until it is sure to receive the next meal. Your body is designed to miraculously survive for days from conserving energy in this manner. It conserves energy using two tactics:

1. The body stores energy as fat when food arrives, just in case more shortages occur. It remembers how bad it was last time it had to go without fuel.

2. The body decreases how much energy it spends, so that it will have enough energy to seek more food. It's like a signal that says, "Hey...slow that metabolism down for a while, until things get back to normal!"

These mechanism will work beautifully if a natural disaster occurs or if we somehow sink into a national food shortage. But it wreaks havoc when we are trying to squeeze into a pair of skinny jeans.

Metabolism has two basic states: the catabolic state and the anabolic state. Catabolism is when your body is breaking down muscle. Anabolism is when your body is building muscle. Going for many hours without food can put your body in to a catabolic state, depending how much protein had been eaten in the last meal.

Perhaps the most likely catabolic state comes after skipping breakfast. You go 8 hours without eating while in bed, but then you don't eat breakfast--even though the point of breakfast is literally to break the fast.

In other words, you eat dinner at 7 pm. You go to bed and get up. You skip breakfast and just have lunch the following day at 12 noon. That's a whopping 17 hours without eating! Even a mid-morning snack at 10 am would put you at 15 hours without eating. It's a double-whammy. Not only does your body begin feeding off your muscle for energy (cannibalizing itself), but it also begins hoarding fat.

In a 2004-2006 Australian research study[1], 2184 participants journaled their diets daily, with specific notation on whether they had eaten breakfast or not. Those who skipped breakfast were found to have larger waist circumferences (bigger bellies), and higher fasting insulin.

Low-calorie, low-fat dieting only aggravates the problem. When you try to use a low-calorie diet, you may just end up burning through muscle and storing fat. Dieting will not only trigger the fat-hoarding, but will slow your metabolic rate as well.

You may have heard fitness trainers use the word, "metabolic rate." The metabolic rate is the number of calories you would burn if you were at rest. It is how much energy you expend when you are not working out. If you think about it, you want to burn calories when you get out of the gym, not only when you're there. The treadmill is just a machine that counts calories while you are there, but the real magic happens when you are not running on it.

Another contributor to the hoarding of fat is the lack of fat intake. When you go on a fat-free or low-fat diet, your body says, "There will be no more fat coming. Hold on to that fat!"

When we eat good fats, we create movement which stimulates abdominal fat. Your old fat is stagnantly resting and needs to be urged to move. Stimulation is good. Stagnation is bad.

Some of the best oils will eliminate stagnation within your body, and the worst oils will "stick," to your body, causing horrific inflammation and cardiovascular disease.

Omega-3 fats are crucial to maintaining health and weight. We'll discuss omega-3 and omega-6 fatty acids in much more detail in Chapter 4. For now, know that one of the major problems with eating processed food is that the worst oils are commonly used—processed omega-6 oils. Most Western diets splurge on omega-6 foods like there's no tomorrow.

We need to eat as much omega-3 fats as possible to balance out our bad tendency to eat omega-6 fats. The omega-6 heavy-hitters are sunflower oil, canola oil, soybean oil, safflower oil, and anything you see labeled "vegetable oil" or "shortening." Stop putting these factory oils in to your cart. You'll find out why you need to avoid these oils in Chapter 5.

In a 2013 obesity study[43], scientists gave 6 grams of fish oil to one group and 6 grams of sunflower oil to the other group. Both groups walked 3 times per week for 45 minutes as a form of exercise. At the end of 4 weeks they found that their levels of omega-3 fatty acids, EPA and DHA were higher. Then they measured again after 8 weeks. They found a significant reduction in weight of the omega-3 fish oil group.

If you eat out often, you are most likely eating heavily processed food. You won't be able to control the type of oil you take in, nor the amount of oil. Find foods which you can prepare quickly at home. You don't always need to make cooking fancy. Trying to follow recipes from famous television chefs can lead to a sense of feeling overwhelmed in the kitchen. Often times, gourmet chefs are aimed at impressing others with their exotic culinary skills, rather than actually showing us how to make basic, everyday food. Daily cooking does not need to be a big project.

Prepare simple foods, and make them in abundance so that you'll have food for a couple days. Go raw sometimes—it's quicker. Get a slow cooker with a delay timer. Then you will be able to eat at home more often. If you are stretched for time one day, shop at the deli/hot foods section of the health food market. Many health food markets carry to-go-meals with the exact ingredients listed. Some even have seating areas. However, eating prepared foods from health food stores can be pricey, so you may want to use this option only when you need to order food out.

Read the following list. Limit foods from the "Bad Fats" list, and eat from foods from the "Good Fats" list daily.

Bad Fats:

- o   Margarine
- o   Vegetable shortening
- o   Vegetable oil
- o   Hydrogenated fats
- o   Canola oil
- o   Sunflower oil
- o   Soybean oil
- o   Corn oil
- o   Safflower oil
- o   Cheese fat (from a soy or corn-fed cow)
- o   Milk & cream fat (from a soy or corn fed cow)
- o   Animal fat/lard (unless from grass-fed source)
- o   Trans-fats

Good Fats:

- Nut fats
- Seed fats
- Hemp oil
- Coconut oil
- Extra-virgin olive oil
- Avocado fat
- Fish oils from salmon, fish roe, mackerel, herring, sardines, and krill
- Tallow (beef fat from grass-fed cow)
- Pastured butter
- Whole pastured milk

Your consumption of fats from the good list will be instrumental to losing belly fat. You will produce more energy, increase muscle mass, and increase your joint health as well. In addition to preparing foods with beneficial fats, you will read about the amazing effect castor oil has on slimming the belly. Castor oil will be key to stimulating trapped fat and toxins within your belly. Once your fat and toxins get moving, your eliminating organs— the skin, kidneys, liver-- will respond and it won't be long before you are enjoying your new flat belly.

Consuming good fats is not simply a healthy option to choose on a whim instead of eating the bad fats. It is not like choosing the whole wheat option at Subway because the whole wheat 6-inch is better for you than white one.

Eating good fats is essential to health and losing fat. It's a must. Get it in! There are healthy folks out there who are adding coconut oil to morning smoothies by the spoonful, just to make sure they get it in. And you too must be diligent about your consumption of the good fats. Add them to everything you eat. It is this consumption of healthy fats which may prevent a heart attack, which will give your skin and hair a beautiful glow, and which will allow you to slip into a pair of jeans without heaving.

Mary G. Enig, Ph.D., a nutritionist and researcher, spent a lifetime researching fats, cholesterol, and heart disease. She warned about the dangers of margarine and trans-fats in 1992, long before it was popular do so, and later pushed for labeling of trans-fats on food products. She strongly advocated the healthy consumption of coconut oil and butter. She maintained that coconut oil did not contribute to cardiovascular disease, and did not contribute to cholesterol in the arteries. Her research is always heavily loaded with solid scientific evidence.

Dr. Enig referred to one particular study in which the diets of Sri Lankans were studied by Dr. Kaunitz and Dr. Dayrit. They said that when the Sri Lankans moved from their home island to New Zealand, they switched oils, and began eating corn oil instead of coconut oil. Their cholesterol changed dramatically, for the worse. Their "bad" cholesterol, LDL did go down 23.8%. But their "good" cholesterol, HDL went down as well, by 41.4%. It created an unfavorable ratio that could eventually lead to the unhealthy depositing of cholesterol on artery walls, a condition known as atherosclerosis. Atherosclerosis, is the build-up of plaque on artery walls which can lead to heart disease if arteries continue to narrow and harden.

Your good fat intake should be at least 30% of your entire daily intake.

All snacks and meals should include fats from the good list. The end of the chapter will provide meal tips and snacks to help you along the way.

The Fat-Free Decade

Many of us that have lived through the '80s are so traumatized by the fat-free-craze that we cannot even wrap our heads around the idea that you need to eat fat in order to lose fat.

Capitalism is great until it ends up in your kitchen cupboard. America was introduced to all kinds of products, from fat-free chips to fat-free cakes during the '80s. The fat was replaced by chemicals to create an "edible" product. Fat-free product still lingers in the supermarket aisles. You can still see food-like substances like, "Light Sour Cream." Even some baked potato chips are fully doused with chemicals. Make a habit out of scanning ingredient lists of processed food. Place it back on the shelf for the next sucker if the list is too long.

The other trickery that happened during the fat-free decade was that manufacturers snatched fat away, but then loaded the products with sugar! The '80s introduced sugar as way to steer clear of fat. Even fat-free jelly beans made the cut.

Sugar is the one ingredient that single-handedly destroys the human body. It is by far the biggest culprit of diseases such as:

o   Cancer
o   Diabetes
o   Heart Disease

And causes problems such as:

o   Belly Fat
o   Insulin Resistance
o   High Blood Pressure
o   Arterial Wall Plaque
o   High Cholesterol

- o High Triglycerides
- o Weakened Immune System

The health food industry has exploited the heck out of sugar as well, arriving just in time with products like agave syrup and evaporated cane juice. These processed products cause as much damage as sugar itself. The only difference is that you are not eating bleached, GMO granules. But you are eating sugar, nonetheless. "Natural" agave syrup is nearly as dangerous as high-fructose corn syrup.

The latest "gluten-free" craze has people munching on bags of sugar-laden gluten- free cookies, cheesy gluten-free pizza, and gluten-free brownies. Gluten-free products allow people to feel better about the processed crap they eat. And people pay big money to feel that way too.

Even more ironic are the new Paleo Diet food products. The Paleo Diet, which is supposed to resemble the way cavemen ate during Lower Paleolithic times, has manufacturers scurrying to invent Paleo product. Now you'll find Paleo bars, Paleo protein powders, and Paleo crackers all wrapped up in plastic, just like any good caveman would eat it. A couple of Paleo products even contain added sugar, in the form of "dextrose."

Recent evidence suggests that sugar may be far more addictive than a pack of cigarettes or crack cocaine. Everyone treats cigarettes and crack cocaine with caution, and everyone regards these substances as highly toxic.

Sugar addiction, or "sweet tooth," on the other hand, is treated with a big bowl of ice cream. Sugar, the silent killer, is accepted and welcomed within society. You have friends, neighbors, and strangers serving it to you as a gesture of kindness. I once had a woman feel sorry for my children because I didn't want to bring them home a mega-pack of donuts that was left over from a work meeting.

Whoa whoa, back up. What's wrong with agave? Agave contains about 85% fructose, making its content higher than sugar. (Sugar is about 50% fructose, 50% glucose.)

Agave is straight-up high in fructose. Fructose sounds like it could be good, doesn't it? It's got the "fru," at least.

Indeed, whole fruits are very good for you, but processing and refining the heck out of their sugar is not. When you eat too much fructose, the liver gets overloaded and starts turning the fructose into fat.

In a 2011 research study[2] where rats ate a high-fat, low-fructose diet, researchers found that they were able to prevent and reverse leptin resistance. Leptin is known for helping to control appetite by binding to receptors in the brain. It also increases sympathetic nervous system activity, stimulating fat to burn energy. Leptin resistance is a condition where the body may have enough of the hormone, Leptin, but it is simply not responding to it. The study is essentially claiming that if you lower sugar intake, your body will work in unison with your leptin hormone, and you'll be less likely to overeat.

In 1989, The American Journal of Clinical Nutrition[3] published a study saying that triglyceride levels (fat) rose when rats were fed fructose. Forget about fat making you fat...its sugar that provides the yellow brick road to belly fat.

You've got to get off that sugar kick. Your life depends on it. Back away from the following sweeteners:

- o Sugar
- o Sucrose
- o Sucralose
- o Evaporated Cane Juice

- o Dextrose
- o Agave
- o Aspartame
- o Commercial Honey

Commercial honey means that the honey has been heated much higher than 95 degrees Fahrenheit or 35 degrees Celsius in order to pasteurize it. Some "natural" beekeepers even get scared about natural bacteria and microwave honey before canning it! Yikes! That's like nuking a cucumber. Honey has living enzymes, but it also has anti-bacterial properties that make it safe for us to eat. It is only unsafe for babies.

Honey is kind of like our beautifully delicate olive, hemp, and flax oils. If you heat them, you not only destroy their healing abilities, but you transform them into something unhealthy. The filtration process also filters good enzymes out of honey.

If you really want to have good honey, look for honey which is local to your region, and which is thick and unclear. It may also say, "raw", but not all beekeepers are familiar with this popular, new term. Some have just always done it that way, and haven't put on a label appealing to the new generation of raw foodies. It's worth it to ask the beekeeper to what extent he processes his honey. If you find a good honey, you get to have your sweet, and your nutrition too.

Also keep stevia on hand. If you crave something sweet, get your butt in to the kitchen and bake it yourself. Stevia is safe and all-natural. It will help you sweeten your coffee, tea, and teriyaki sauce. If you need to indulge in baked treats occasionally, substitute Stevia for the sugar. Stevia makes cookies and cakes far less dangerous.

We didn't know what to eat in the '80s. We just knew that fat was the enemy. All fat was shunned. That's when canola oil rolled in, telling us all the things we wanted to hear. By the '90s, companies managed to convince us that big vats of canola oil was the way to go. Yes, oil was okay, as long as it was canola.

My family kept a big Costco bottle of canola oil under the sink for many years. There are still households across America who believe they are being healthy by frying fish in canola oil instead of Crisco Vegetable Shortening. Crisco themselves even started selling their version of the pretty canola oil. When people see "clear," they see "health," and off they go with their cute carcinogenic oil in their shopping baskets.

90% of canola oil comes from a genetically modified Rapeseed plant. Lovely name. The oil is extracted from the plant using a chemical called Hexane. The oil then goes through an extensive refining process which involves bleaching and heating omega-3 fats. Omega-3 fats are wonderful until you add high heat. Then the oil becomes rancid and carcinogenic.

Omega-3 Fats + High Heat = Trans-Fats, aka Partially Hydrogenated Oil

Heating omega-3 oils can cause cancer, because they release free radicals into your body. Even when you heat a healthy oil like extra-virgin olive oil, you are creating a carcinogenic trans-fat factory, right there in your own kitchen.

Mega health food store, Whole Foods is currently being shunned by some health foodies for preparing its hot deli foods with canola oil. Indeed the canola oil ingredient puzzles many who scan the ingredient labels placed above the hot food trays.

However, Whole Foods claims they use a non-GMO canola and that it is expeller-pressed—not extracted with Hexane. It's probably okay to trust Whole Foods on this one, and enjoy their meals on occasion.

However, you'll want to steer clear of eating this oil on the daily basis, and don't even think about ruining your food pantry with a big vat of the stuff. Sabotaging your health with daily doses of carcinogenic canola oil is the last thing you want to do anyway. If you are going to indulge, at least give yourself something delicious, like a hunk of chocolate, or a slice of pizza. You only have a limited number of cheat cards to pull out during the month. Don't waste them on canola oil. Make your own treats using coconut oil. Use it for cooking at high temperatures, and reap the rewards that fly your way.

How Much Fat to Eat to Lose Weight

Now that we have dispelled some of the fat phobias, we can discuss how much fat to eat in order to help shed fat. Obviously you don't want to eat tons of fat, because then your body will be mostly comprised of fat. Your daily intake of fat should be roughly 30% of total daily calorie intake to lose weight. The term, "weight loss," or "lose weight," will be used throughout this book and will always mean "fat loss." By using a combination of healthy fats and proteins in your kitchen, you can effectively lose weight.

Note that the quality of fat is of upmost importance. If you eat poor fats, you are at risk for disease and you will probably be fat as well. The 30% fat is not a free-for-all fat fest. It is simply a guideline to use. If you indulge in the wrong oils, or you eat far too much of the right oils, your results will not be pretty.

Fats have traditionally been divided into two categories---saturated fat and unsaturated fat. The major saturated fat players are animal fat (including dairy) and coconut oil. Yes, the healthy coconut oil.

We used to believe that coconut oil was bad because it contained saturated fat. However, recent research has shown exactly the opposite. Saturated fat does not cause cardiovascular disease. Further, the type of saturated fat that coconut oil contains is much different from the long chain type that comes from animal fat. Coconut oil contains medium chain fatty acids. Coconut fat is metabolized by the body much differently than animal fat.

Coconut oil is less likely to be stored as body fat because the fat is absorbed from the digestive tract and used by the liver for energy. It also helps increase your metabolism and supports insulin sensitivity. You want that support.

To benefit from coconut oil, start by consuming 1 tablespoon daily. You can consume up to 3 tablespoons each day, but it is safest to begin your coconut oil routine slowly. You will see an increase in metabolism, along with an increase in bowel movements. If you take too much too soon, you may even see loose stools. So take it easy and start with 1 tablespoon daily until you feel comfortable moving to 2 tablespoons.

Once coconut oil is regularly consumed, most people notice a difference in:

- o Metabolism
- o Digestion
- o Energy Level
- o Blood Circulation

Coconut oil simply gets everything to flow better. When your blood flow increases, you increase the amount of oxygen supplied to your cells. This in turn increases your metabolism, and the way you process food. The damage that margarine and canola oil do to your digestion (heartburn, acid reflux, bloating) are absent with coconut oil.

Less Gas=More Flat

The medium chain fatty acids in coconut oil are:

o Caprylic Acid
o Capric Acid
o Lauric Acid

In a 2003 study[4] of 19 overweight men, scientists found that when the participants ate a diet rich in medium chain fatty acids (like the ones in coconut oil) for 4 weeks, they exhibited an increase in energy expenditure and diminished fat. Subsequently, they lost weight by eating medium-chain fats.

Study after study shows that medium chain fatty acids increase energy and help you lose fat.

In another study[5], scientists compared a diet of medium chain oils, caprylic acid and capric acid to a diet of beef tallow in 27 overweight women. The women were fed the diets on site, and tested after 27 days. The women who ate the medium chain fats increased fat oxidation and energy expenditure. This study suggests that substituting medium chain fats like coconut oil for long-chain fats like beef tallow, increases weight loss.

Medium chain fatty acids are used in both medications and in food processing because they are:

o   Anti-Bacterial

o   Anti-Fungal

o   Anti-Viral

o   Anti-Parasitic

These fats help prevent and cure infectious disease, so naturally they are used in medicine and food processing to help reduce spoilage. The medium chain fatty acids in coconut oil are even known to help protect babies from microbial bacteria, so it's a good idea for pregnant and nursing mothers to supplement with coconut oil.

How Much Protein to Eat

Any advice on losing belly fat would be incomplete if it did not stress the importance of eating protein. In addition to making sure you have enough fat to lose fat, pay close attention to your protein intake.

The amount of protein you should eat will depend on how hard you work out. If you lift weights and build muscle, you need more protein. If you sit around a lot, you need much less.

You also need to continue to adjust protein levels according to your level of activity. If you sat on your behind last month, but managed to get to the gym a lot more this month, raise your protein intake.

Maybe you worked out hard last month, but this month you take a 7-day vacation, and then slowly ease back in to the gym. Lower your protein until you are back in to the swing of things. Life circumstances like moving, divorce, or changing work schedules can change your need for protein. Even the kids' soccer schedule can mess up your gym time.

Some people make the grave mistake of continuing to eat like they did when they were a teenager on the softball team, or when they were training for a particular running event.

Guys are notorious for wolfing down an obscene amount of meat, but somehow forgetting to make it into the gym with you. They used to hit it heavy back in the day, so they know how important protein is. But they somehow can't find their shoes when it's actually time to go to the gym. Their excess protein will eventually become stored fat, so they need to cut back until they are ready to go and lift. Of course not all guys are like this, but you get the picture.

Evaluate your protein needs frequently, and then raise or lower them to keep up with whatever you are doing. See below to figure your current daily protein needs:

> Sedentary 150-lb Woman (sitting around way too much, or physically unable to walk): Consume 46-54 grams protein per day.
> Lightly Active 150-lb Woman (walking daily): Consume 54-70 grams protein per day.
> Active 150-lb Woman (moderately working out): Consume 70-100 grams protein per day.
> Very Active 150lb Woman (building muscle, intense athletic exertion): Consume 100-120 grams of protein per day.

Protein should account for 35% of your caloric intake everyday if you want to lose fat and gain muscle. Good fats should account for at least 30%. The remaining 35% of your daily intake can be fibrous carbs. Fibrous carbs include mostly veggies and some fruit. Grains are optional. Don't go crazy with them, but if you choose to include them, make sure they are from a whole source. Whole wheat bread and whole wheat pasta are much more processed than potatoes, oats, and rice.

Coupling carbs with protein will prevent your insulin from spiking. When your insulin spikes, your blood glucose also rises and your body craves more food to soothe the situation. Always eat carbs with protein. This can be as easy as popping a hard-boiled egg in your mouth before you eat that pasta meal.

Remember, many proteins contain the bad kind of saturated fat. Saturated fat from corn or soy-fed pigs, corn-fed chickens, and grain-fed cows is unhealthy. The meat is too. Choose from the following good protein list:

Good Proteins:

- Chicken Breast
- Salmon
- 2 Egg White + 1 Whole Egg
- Tuna
- Herring
- Mackerel
- Whey Protein Powder
- Hemp Protein Powder
- Pea Protein Powder
- Vegan Protein Power Blend
- Egg White Protein Powder
- Grass-Fed Whey Protein Powder
- Grass-Fed Beef
- Beans (no soy)

In a 2012 obesity study called, "Quality Protein is Inversely Related with Abdominal Fat[6]," scientists measured the protein, fat and carbohydrates of 27 men and women. They found that the intake of quality (protein containing essential amino acids) protein during the day was inversely related to how much central abdominal fat (belly fat) the participants had when measured during a 24-hour period. They concluded that quality protein has a strong correlation to abdominal fat and plays an important role.

In plain Engrish: Eat protein in every meal for less belly fat.

Beauty comes from within, sure. But what about outer beauty? The physical attributes you consider to be beautiful about a person are largely made up of proteins. Protein is largely responsible for building skin, hair, and muscle. Healthy hair which does not break easily is made of protein. A toned body which is not dimpled with cellulite will also contain a good amount of protein.

When we work out hard, we use the body strenuously. The body needs protein to keep up with the amount of work we are giving it. You know you need to exercise at least 3 times per week to maintain health. But are you getting enough lean protein? As a rule, the more you work out, the more protein you need to eat. Eat protein before and after workouts. Eat it at every meal too.

If you are not consuming protein, your body will seek protein from somewhere in your body and apply it to wherever it sees fit. Your body will eventually begin to cannibalize itself. It will take protein from wherever it can get it---your leg, your tricep, your back. And you will be left with some jiggily mass of fat. If you've been going to the gym for a while and you are still jiggily, or are experiencing a plateau, try adding more protein to your diet. Protein will help burn fat and increase muscle.

You will have moments when your body wants to use protein to repair the small injuries that may happen throughout the course of a week, month, or year. It could be that you cut your finger while cooking and new skin needs to be built. It could be that you strained your hamstring and now your muscle tissue needs to be reconstructed. Even just being generally sore from working out hard is an event that the body will need to repair. Sure the soreness will go away after a couple days, but shouldn't you be helping out by supplying it with enough amino acids to complete the task? The body requires amino acids to repair and recover from nearly everything.

Protein is made of about twenty-one amino acids. Nine of these amino acids must be eaten; the body cannot make them on its own. The nine amino acids which must come from a food source are known as essential amino acids.

Nine Essential Amino Acids:

1. Histidine
2. Isoleucine
3. Leucine
4. Lycine
5. Methionine
6. Phenylalanine
7. Threonine
8. Tryptophan
9. Valine

Four non-essential amino acids which your body can make on its own or can make using some of the essential amino acids are:

10. Alanine

11. Asparagine

12. Aspartic Acid

13. Glutamic Acid

Eight conditional amino acids which become essential and needed if you are stressed, sick, or workout hard are:

14. Arginine

15. Cysteine

16. Glutamine

17. Glycine

18. Ornithine

19. Proline

20. Serin

21. Tyrosine

When you see protein powders and workout supplements, you are usually looking at a wide array of both essential and conditional amino acids. Supplementing with conditional amino acids is a good idea if you are placing yourself under a lot of stress with physical labor, or if you are trying to build muscle and lose fat. Making dramatic changes to your body, like getting it to bare heavy weight or completing an hour of intense aerobics is placing stress on your body. Help your body repair itself by consuming enough protein.

It's hard to imagine that someone would choose to not exercise at all, though it does exist. This advice is written for people who are already exercising, but can't get the big belly to flatten. In the rare case that anyone is reading this beauty book and not exercising regularly, please be aware that you will need less protein if you do not workout. Excess protein can be hard on the kidneys, since your body has to eliminate what it does not use. However, if you are indeed reaping the excellent mental and physical benefits of working out—congratulations. Reward your body with protein.

In addition to building and repairing your body, protein also increases metabolism. If you consume enough protein, the rate at which you burn energy will increase while you rest. The rate at which you exert energy while you rest is known as BMR, or Basal Metabolic Rate. In other words, it's the rate at which you burn calories while you are sleeping. BMR slows down for most people as they age. So far, we have already discussed one way to increase BMR--through eating coconut oil. Two other ways to increase BMR is by exercising regularly and by consuming protein regularly. Eating protein will increase your metabolism so that you can continue burning fat long after you step off the treadmill. You want this. It means you'll wake up skinnier.

Eating protein will also stabilize blood sugar, bypassing fat mode. The hoarding of fat is not only attributed to lack of healthy fat consumption, but is also related to not eating enough protein. The idea is to increase insulin sensitivity and to decrease insulin resistance.

Insulin is a hormone which regulates metabolism and blood sugar. It either:

> Removes excess glucose (a type of sugar) and stores it in the liver and muscles as glycogen, OR
> Stores it as adipose fat (body fat) and triglycerides

The best approach is to create an insulin sensitive environment to ensure the insulin is always storing in the muscles and liver. A high-carb or sugary meal will most likely blow the roof off your blood sugar levels, and cause your insulin to store fat.

In a research study of women aged 18-55[7], scientists found that the more protein the women ate for breakfast, the less their glucose and insulin spiked. Each woman got a meal consisting of either: a. Pancakes with 3 grams of protein b. Egg and sausage with 30 grams protein, or c. Egg and sausage with 39 grams protein. All meals contained the same amount of fiber and the same amount of fat. All the women's glucose and insulin levels were measured for four hours following the meal. The women who ate the most protein experienced less blood sugar spikes than the others. The group that consumed 30 grams of protein (group b) had lower spikes than the group who only ate 3 grams of protein.

Protein can help stabilize blood sugar when you have a high-carb item. It's simple:

Always eat carbs with protein

Of course it's best to limit carbs if you are on a fat loss diet. But when you have them, be sure to follow the one simple rule of always eating your carbs with some kind of protein. Many dishes are not traditionally served with protein. Pizza and beer, pasta with pesto, and cheese enchiladas are all examples of meals that we tend to eat without protein. Desserts do not contain any noteworthy protein either. So if you are going to have a dessert, have a piece of chicken or an egg right before. Having the protein right before you indulge will lessen the damage.

You want to avoid triggering the insulin. Think of it like sneaking some friends into the party without insulin noticing. The more insulin notices, the fatter you become. People with insulin resistance will have to shell out a ton of insulin from their pancreas to keep their blood sugar stable. Insulin resistance is bad. Insulin sensitivity is good.

You may find it easy to boil several eggs and refrigerate them during the week, so that you can pop one into your mouth as needed. Two egg yolks per day is ideal. If you eat a lot of eggs every day, make sure they are mostly egg whites, along with one or two whole eggs.

If your body becomes insulin resistant, you will probably develop a lot of fat in the mid-section. Here's how to create an insulin sensitive body which will cut belly fat:

1. Eat a moderately high protein diet
2. Exercise regularly, especially with weights
3. Sleep 7-9 hours daily
4. Eat more omega-3 Fatty Acids
5. Eat less omega-6 Fatty Acids
6. Eat all meals, especially breakfast
7. Eat whole, real foods—no processed crap
8. Always eat any carbs with protein
9. Relax. Stop stressing out

Creating an insulin sensitive body will keep glucose levels steady and help cut belly fat.

Eating a protein breakfast could also help you avoid snacking later on in the day too. In a study of 18-20 year olds[8], a team of University of Missouri researchers found that when the girls ate a high-protein breakfast, they were less likely to snack during the day and evening.

The girls were split in to three groups. The first group had no breakfast. The second group had lean beef and eggs (whatever...maybe Vegas-style steak and eggs), while the third group had boxed cereal. They then studied the girls' brain signals in an MRI scan. As you might have guessed, the first group was a hungry bunch of little women.

The ones who ate the most protein in the morning had the most satiety, or fullness. Heather J. Leidy and her team of researchers state that eating a high protein breakfast, "reduces pre-lunch neural activation in brain regions that control food motivation/reward." Hmmm...I'll take some reduction in my pre-lunch neural activation too.

Vegans and Vegetarians—How to Get it In

For to-go snacks, nuts can't be beat. They're handy, snacky, nutritious, and convenient. They have copious amounts of good fats and minerals. They don't really belong in the protein arena though. They have just enough protein to sustain you until the next meal, but they shouldn't be the meal. When you are trying to meet the day's requirement, it is best to eat from lean, high-protein sources. Nuts, yogurt, and milk do contain protein, but they contain far too little protein, and far too much of the other nutrients to make it an actual protein source. You would have to consume bags and bags of nuts in order to meet protein requirements. You'll get fat if you eat too many of these little guys. When you eat protein, choose dense protein from the protein list.

Soy is not included on the list because of its tendency to mimic estrogen in both female and male bodies. It is probably okay to consume soy once or twice per week, but eating soy on the daily or regular basis can create hormone imbalance. Anyone who has a hormone imbalance can tell you that it makes maintaining a fit body very difficult. Go to the doctor and check it out. A doctor can do a blood or urine test to see if your hormones are in balance. There's also a great online hormone quiz[9], along with an at-home saliva test. The site is run by Dr. John Lee out of California, and he is very good at explaining hormones, for those of us that didn't make it in to Harvard.

An estrogen-dominant body will contain a lot of fat on the belly, as well as on the back and butt. No, not the hot Brazil butt. The dimpled, cellulite-style butt. An overabundance of estrogen will cause cellulite. Not only does overuse of soy cause fat storage and cellulite, but it furthers your risk of fibroids and breast cancer. The majority of soy is processed and contains GMO's in addition to its tendency to mimic estrogen.

Here is a quote taken directly from the Weston A. Price Foundation on the dangers of this phytoestrogen:

"

Confused About Soy?–Soy Dangers Summarized

> ➢ High levels of phytic acid in soy reduce assimilation of calcium, magnesium, copper, iron and zinc. Phytic acid in soy is not neutralized by ordinary preparation methods such as soaking, sprouting and long, slow cooking. High phytate diets have caused growth problems in children.
> ➢ Trypsin inhibitors in soy interfere with protein digestion and may cause pancreatic disorders. In test animals soy containing trypsin inhibitors caused stunted growth.
> ➢ Soy phytoestrogens disrupt endocrine function and have the potential to cause infertility and to promote breast cancer in adult women.

➢ Soy phytoestrogens are potent antithyroid agents that cause hypothyroidism and may cause thyroid cancer. In infants, consumption of soy formula has been linked to autoimmune thyroid disease.

➢ Vitamin B12 analogs in soy are not absorbed and actually increase the body's requirement for B12.

➢ Soy foods increase the body's requirement for vitamin D.

➢ Fragile proteins are denatured during high temperature processing to make soy protein isolate and textured vegetable protein.

➢ Processing of soy protein results in the formation of toxic lysinoalanine and highly carcinogenic nitrosamines.

➢ Free glutamic acid or MSG, a potent neurotoxin, is formed during soy food processing and additional amounts are added to many soy foods.

➢ Soy foods contain high levels of aluminum which is toxic to the nervous system and the kidneys."

The foundation website[10] has a wealth of studies and in-depth information about the effects of soy. If you're in America, soy or corn can sneak in to anything you touch. Either stick to real food, or scrutinize ingredient labels.

It's quite possible to be vegan and meet your daily protein requirements, even if you only prepare foods with soy very occasionally, and do not rely on it as a daily protein source. Simply Google "Vegan Bodybuilders" and you will see some examples of having beautiful lean muscle mass without consuming animals.

However, if are going to be vegan, you must be extremely diligent about your diet. Eating processed Tofu Pups everyday will make you unhealthy, and should not be considered as "plant-based." or "health food." Don't cram a bunch of Oreos into your mouth just because you heard they're vegan.

No Meat Athlete[11] is a great resource for vegans and vegetarians. The website is hip to the fact that loading up on soy doesn't work. Neither is there a bunch of processed vegan foods on the site. A real-food approach is what everyone needs. Real proteins. Real fats. Real veggies.

It's a lot easier to get protein when you are vegetarian (as opposed to vegan), because you eat eggs and whey. But the new vegan protein powders are constantly improving. It's getting easier than ever to maintain the vegan lifestyle. True Nutrition out of San Diego and My Protein out of England make excellent soy-free, vegan protein powders. Both shops have "custom-made" powders, where you control the sweetener. It's kind of cool to have the vegan powders whether you are vegan or not. They will help you eat a well-balanced diet. And... just cause hemp is awesome too. Having too much of anything is usually not good for you. Mix it up with a little vegan power.

You can get unsweetened protein powder and put it in foods other than just smoothies. Protein powders blend beautifully into vegetable soups. They have custom egg white powder as well, if you are not vegan, but are lactose-intolerant. Egg white powder can be blended with cauliflower and broth to make a creamy protein soup. It works with butternut squash soup as well. Just boil the ingredients, spoon them to a blender, and add the protein powder, some coconut oil, and salt or bouillon. If you have a Vitamix blender, you know what to do. Work your magic.

Sometimes being vegan or raw vegan can be a salvation. It can clear the mind and body of conflict and disease. But it can also be a hindrance if you are not extra careful about getting protein and good fat. Your body knows what to do. Listen to it. If your body calls for no meat, then so be it. Just don't let veganism turn you into a factory-processed blob of man-made foods.

When people claim that vegetarians live longer, they're not referring to the ones eating processed vegan chick'n product every day. Stick to real food on your plant-based diet. Whatever the case may be, trust in your body and your cravings...unless the craving are chips and Oreos. Don't trust those.

Meals and Snacks: How to Get it In

Now that you know abs are made in the kitchen, you might be wondering, what do I eat? Here are some guidelines to eat the right foods to help you flatten that belly:

Use extra-virgin coconut when cooking and extra-virgin olive oil when preparing salads or cold dishes. Dishes that taste great with coconut oil include:

Breakfasts:

Cereals and breads do not usually make good breakfasts, despite strong cultural tradition. They create insulin resistance first thing in the morning, and most cereals are filled with dyes, gmo's, sugar, and other crap you don't need. Oats is a good non-processed grain option, and it comes with a respectable amount of fiber. If you must eat cereal or bread for breakfast, remember to eat it some egg or other protein. Otherwise, try either of these two breakfasts to fill your stomach and control blood sugar. Eating a high protein breakfast will jumpstart your metabolism and reduce cravings throughout the day.

Scrambled Eggs for Two

2 whole eggs
4 egg whites
¼ c coconut milk
½ tablespoon coconut oil
Dash sea salt

Break eggs in to medium-sized bowl. Add coconut milk and salt. Beat eggs with electric beater for 15 seconds or whisk by hand 30 seconds. Heat coconut oil on medium heat. Add eggs and cook for 3-5 minutes. Do not brown eggs. Eat sometimes with salsa or guacamole to switch it up.

Piña Colada Smoothie, Serves One

1 cup coconut milk
1 1-inch thick slice pineapple
1 banana
1 handful washed spinach or kale
1 tablespoon coconut oil
2 tablespoons raw pumpkin seeds
2 tablespoons raw sunflower seeds
1 scoop protein powder of choice

Place everything in blender and blend. Pour into large glass or Mason jar. Enjoy!

Lunches and Dinners

Remember, you can add a tablespoon of extra-virgin coconut oil into virtually everything you make. Try these dishes out. All dishes serve 3-4 people. The brown rice will probably last you more days, depending on how many people are eating.

Seared Chicken Breast

4 boneless, skinless chicken breasts
1 tablespoon extra-virgin coconut oil
Sea Salt & Pepper

Rinse and thoroughly pat chicken dry with paper towels. Heat 1 tablespoon of coconut oil in pan, preferably cast iron. Place chicken in pan and sprinkle/grind a little salt and pepper on each breast. After about 3 minutes, check brownness. If golden brown, flip with tongs or spatula and brown other side. Serve hot with salad and brown or white rice.

Seared Grass-Fed Steak

1 lb. grass-fed New York steak
1 tablespoon extra-virgin coconut oil
Sea Salt & Pepper

Rinse and thoroughly pat steak dry with paper towels. Cut steak into 4 equal portions. Heat 1 tablespoon of coconut oil in pan, preferably cast iron. Place steaks in pan and sprinkle/grind a little salt and pepper on each breast. After about 3-5 minutes, check brownness. If golden brown, flip with tongs or spatula and brown other side. Serve hot with salad and brown or white rice.

Steamed Salmon

1 lb Alaskan salmon

1 tablespoon extra-virgin coconut oil

Stove or electric steamer

Rinse salmon and slice into to 4 equal portions. Steam 10 minutes. With spoon or butter knife, spread coconut oil on to Salmon. Serve hot with herbed boiled potatoes and steamed broccoli.

Slow Cooker Red Beans

½ lb. red beans

Water

½ green pepper, finely chopped

½ c onion, finely chopped

3 cloves garlic, minced

1 stalk celery, finely chopped

½ tablespoon paprika

Pepper

Sea Salt

2 tablespoons coconut oil

2 teaspoons Veggie or Chicken Better than Bouillon or other brand bouillon.

Soak red beans overnight. Next day, place red beans, green pepper, onion, celery, garlic, paprika, bay leaf, and pepper in slow cooker. Do not add salt. Add water to cover. Cook 8 hours on low in slow cooker. At the end, ladle out as much of cooking water as possible. Discard cooking water. Add bouillon and coconut oil. If salt is needed, add to taste.

Brown Rice

2 rice cooker sized cups of brown rice
Rice cooker
1 tablespoon coconut oil
¼ cup onion, chopped
2 cloves garlic, minced
Sea Salt
¼ teaspoon turmeric, optional

Rinse 2 rice cooker cups of brown rice under cold water in colander. Add water to the appropriate fill line. Add coconut oil, onion, and garlic. Add turmeric (optional). Cook brown rice according to rice cooker manufacturer instructions. Or bring to a boil, then simmer on low heat 25 minutes, or until rice is soft.

Lime-Olive Oil Salad Dressing

¼ cup lime juice
¼ cup extra-virgin olive oil
1 tablespoon Dijon mustard
2 cloves garlic, chopped
Sea Salt to taste

Combine everything in small jar. Close lid and shake. Add sea salt to taste. Spoon dressing onto salad.

Chapter Summary

1. Protein increases metabolism and helps slim the belly.

2. You need to eat fat in order to lose fat. Essential fatty acids (from good oils) are as important as essential amino acids (from good protein).

3. Sugar sucks everything good out of your body. Go for raw honey or stevia instead.

Chapter Two

Castor Oil—The Crazy Healing Oil

Losing the Belly

What's in there, and why doesn't it go away?

It's not all fat—at least, not the kind you trim off a steak. It is various things--it may be pus, inflamed intestines, gas, parasites, mucous, and trapped food. You may even have some Candida overgrowth thrown into the mix.

According to the Society of Interventional Radiology[12], 20-40% of women 35 years and older have fibroids. Fibroids are non-cancerous tumors that grow in the uterus. If you are black, that number is more like 50%. If you over the age of 50, the number is 20-80%, according to the Office on Women's Health at the U.S. Department of Health and Human Services[13]. An ovarian cyst is a fluid-filled sac on the ovary.

It's quite common to have fibroids and/or cysts. It's just taboo to talk about anything going on down there. You'll never hear anyone bring it up over crumpets and tea. We just walk around thinking we are the only ones with an abnormal situation. Fibroids and ovarian cysts only cause symptoms in 25% of women that have them. Most women don't even know they have them. It would take an ultrasound to know for certain.

If you have any abdominal inflammation and/or distress, you will most likely benefit from castor oil. Castor oil should be used in conjunction with doctor visits.

You'll need to get a diagnosis of what kind of cysts you have in order to figure out a plan of attack. Some cysts develop from hormonal imbalance.

Having a belly is not a sign of laziness. There's plenty of people who work hard, or exercise regularly that still have a belly. Is that you? It was certainly me.

My Success with Castor Oil

I worked out and worked out, yet I still had this big belly. It didn't even seem affected by exercise. It had everything to do with food. If I only had soup or a protein shake for dinner, I could get it a little flatter the following day. But in general, my belly did not reflect how much I cared about my health. I simply didn't look like anyone who went to the gym, yet I was in there working it hard every single day!

I tried cleanse after cleanse to reduce my gut. I also did acupuncture performed by a traditional Chinese doctor. On the very first visit, she made a list of "no" foods and "yes" foods and told me in broken English to follow it for one year. This was incredibly helpful. She said not to eat peanut butter, sugar, beans, coffee, and crackers. Good thing she did not know about my fetish for chips.

Not eating peanut butter was a big shocker. At the time, I had begun a new vegan diet, and had just polished off a peanut butter and jelly sandwich before walking through her front door.

The girl sitting next to me in the waiting room had the exact same problem, and she couldn't control herself with a jar of peanut butter either. Peanut butter is like crack to some women.

The no/yes list, along with the acupuncture, eased my lower abdomen inflammation. But I still had that belly.

I also visited a great naturopath in town, where I was diagnosed with pelvic congestion. She described the problem plaguing many of today's women: We sit at our desks all day long and our pelvises become like bowls. All of the toxins we ingest everyday--through our food, through the air, through the beverages we drink—all come to sit in this bowl of ours. This bowl becomes congested and overfilled with toxins throughout time. After years of this, the reproductive system cannot flow and function properly. Eggs cannot be delivered timely, and monthly periods don't arrive, most often delayed due to low visibility on the runways.

The inflammation subsided with the guidance of these wonderful natural doctors. But a few years later, it was back with a vengeance. I had developed the same problem again over the holidays. I knew what the culprit was. I was pigging out on too much mashed potatoes, gravy, wine, beer, and pie. I told myself I would stop it all on New Year's Day.

I could feel a knot and pain in my right side growing larger and larger from all my glutinous behavior. I feared the horrendous "appendicitis." Yep...that one illness that I could possibly die from if I didn't do anything right here, right now. My mind imagined the worst. I panicked. I jumped in the car and raided the urgent care clinic. I spilled out my symptoms to the doctor.

I was relieved to hear that I didn't have appendicitis. I learned that it was most likely an ovarian cyst. The doctor said it was a common problem, but that an ultrasound was needed to be sure. She gave me a card to make an appointment at the women's center and sent me home.

I can't remember where I first found out about castor oil. Sometimes information comes flying at me from nowhere at lightning speed. But I decided to try a castor oil pack that night over my belly. IT WORKED WONDERS.

Uhhh, you should probably skip over this next part. I shouldn't be telling you this. If you do end up reading it, try and forget you ever read it, okay? I do not want to be remembered for what I'm about to say.

I had tons of junk coming out of my vajayjay the morning after the first castor oil treatment. Bizarre stuff—things I had never seen before, like clumps and clumps of yellow and white discharge along with clumps of mucous. I was pretty shocked and bewildered. I quickly realized my uterus was cleansing. I practiced the castor oil packs for two more nights. Eventually the clumps lessened, and I got a long-overdue menstrual period.

While I had performed a few colon cleanses, I had never cleansed my uterus before. What a difference it made.

After three nights, my belly was flat. No pus, no gas, no bloating, no hidden mysterious substances inside. I was both laughing and crying to myself out of sheer joy. I couldn't believe how ridiculously cheap, easy, and fast it was to use the castor oil.

I've since used castor oil for everything from moisturizer to varicose veins. It has simplified my life, and made my natural health journey waay more affordable. I don't know about you, but I am sort of a "natural health junkie." I like to try everything and see if it works. Sometimes I'm suckered, and sometimes I'm sold. But one thing's for sure, it costs a pretty penny trying out all the herbs, oils, and supplements. Castor oil takes the cake for being an inexpensive cure-all item. I have it on hand at all times.

Just last week I foolishly cut my hand opening a sharp can, and was bleeding like crazy. Here's what I did:

1. I washed the wound.
2. I swiftly grabbed a paper towel and applied pressure.
3. I applied castor oil, and then applied a bandage. The sting was gone within moments after applying the oil.

Lying.

It was more like this:

1. I curse the can, and look around, dumbfounded. *I will not get blood on any of my new dish towels.*
2. I wash the wound, cover the deep cut with a paper towel and apply pressure.
3. Whimpering now, I run to get Hubby.
4. I dab castor oil on the cut just before Hubby applies a bandage. I cry to Hubby about ruining the can and valuable contents inside can.
5. Hubby states that the hand is more important than the can.
6. Hubby finishes opening the can as I stand back and watch.

Dumb can.

My deep cut then proceeded to heal itself at record speed. I was astonished. It completely healed within one week, pain-free.

Once you discover castor oil, you will love its magical healing power. You will be pleading with the gods for something to happen, just so you can break out some castor oil.

What is Castor Oil and How Does it Benefit the Body?

Castor oil has been used throughout the world for hundreds of centuries. India, Egypt, China, Persia, Rome, and Greece have all been documented to have benefitted from this natural healing oil.

In alternative medicine, castor oil is known to drive impurities away from the body, strengthen the immune system, and assist in lymph flow. The oil is affordable and is used to heal a wide variety of illnesses.

Your body's lymphatic system is your main shield against predators. Lymph cannot easily circulate around your body when the lymphatic system is sluggish. If your lymphatic system is sluggish, you will become susceptible to illness. Castor oil helps lymph circulate, thus increasing your immune response.

Edward Cayce, a clairvoyant healer, shed light on the ancient oil for Americans in the 1930's. Also termed, "Palma Christi," or "Hand of Christ" since the Medieval Times, the oil has been believed to have amazing healing properties. He maintained that the oil worked through energy vibration, by stimulating the nervous system. Here is a list quoted by Cayce in The Oil That Heals by William McGarey[14], of what castor oil does:

"Increases eliminations

Stimulates the liver

Dissolves and removes adhesions

Dissolves and remove lesions

Relieves pain

Releases colon impaction

Reduces nervous

Stimulates the gall bladder

Reduces toxemia

Reduces flatulence

Increases lymphatic circulation

Improves intestinal assimilation

Balances eliminations

Reduces inflammation

Increases relaxation

Dissolves gallstones

Stimulates lacteal duct circulation

Reduces swelling

Stimulates the caecum

Coordinates liver-kidney function

Stimulates organs and glands

The castor oil pack therapy was used by Cayce on people who were diagnosed with the following diseases:

"Aphonia

Cancer

Colitis

Gallstones

Hepatitis

Hookworm

Stenosis of the Duodenum

Neuritis

Lymphitis

Uremia

Parkinson's Disease

Appendicitis

Cholecystitis

Constipation

Gastritis

Hernia

Intestinal Impaction

Stricture of Duodenum

Cirrhosis of Liver

Cerebral Palsy

Sterility

Dr. William McGarey began using castor oil to cure patients of many illnesses, including digestive problems, tumors, and arthritis. He documented the results in his book.

The book was written after 38 years of using castor oil to heal patients. He tells us to simply review the results of the healings of thousands of people. He also notes that the same oil had been used for a wide variety of unrelated conditions.

Castor oil is made from the beans of the Ricinus Communis plant. The beans themselves are toxic because of a compound called Ricin. However, the pressing of the beans renders Ricin inactive and the oil becomes safe for common use.

It is anti-bacterial, anti-fungal, and anti-viral. The oil is also known to help cleanse the body, by helping the lymphatic system to transport and drain toxins. Dr. McGarey states that castor oil enhances the thymus gland, increasing the T-lymphocyte count, and helps eliminate waste from the body. T-lymphocytes are commonly known as white blood cells. These are the good guys. When your body is infected with a virus, it sends these guys in for protection.

Generally, the thymus gland is the largest during childhood, and begins to shrink with age after puberty. The thymus gland is the main organ for the lymphatic system. It helps increase development of white blood cells. The more you are able to support or enhance the function of your thymus gland, the better you will be able to fight and control bacteria and viruses from invading.

Both blood circulation and lymphatic circulation are enhanced when castor oil is applied to the skin. The oil is known to penetrate up to four inches below the surface of the skin. That explains why my finger healed up so quickly.

In a study published in the Journal of Naturopathic Medicine[15], scientists study the effects of "castor oil packs" on 36 healthy men and women. One group was given castor oil packs, and the other group was given paraffin packs.

They covered the umbilical and liver areas for two hours with wool soaked in castor oil. Then they placed a heat pad over the soaked wool.

They drew blood from the participants four times—once before the treatment, another time right before the removal of the treatment, then again seven hours after the removal. The final draw was the following morning, at a full 24 hours since the first draw.

There was not much difference between the participants in the first blood draw. However, the results showed big differences at the third blood draw. They found that the group that had applied castor oil packs had a significant increase in T-11 cells, which they interpreted as a "general boost in the body's specific defense status."

These are the same cells Dr. McGarey wrote about in his book. T-cells are white blood cells which identify and kill virus, bacteria, fungi, and cancer cells. It is said that a person with HIV/AIDS has a lower number of T-cells.

The researchers concluded that castor oil had a beneficial effect on the lymphatic system, and that it enhanced the immune system function.

When shopping for castor oil, buy only hexane-free castor oil, and make sure it is cold-pressed, as heat will disrupt castor oil's fatty acids. The main fatty acid in castor oil, ricinoleic acid, is found nowhere else. It is an unsaturated omega-9 fatty acid that can only be found in castor oil. Wikipedia breaks down castor oil's fatty acid composition as the following:

Ricinoleic Acid	85-95%
Dihydroxystearic Acid	0.7%
Palmitic Acid	1.0%
Stearic Acid	0.5-1%
Oleic Acid	2-6%
Linoleic Acid	1-5%
Linolenic Acid	0.1-1%
Eicosanoic & Other Acids	0.2-0.5%

In addition to being used for medicinal purposes, the oil is used in several industries, including food preservation because of its mold-inhibiting properties. It is used in the cosmetics industry as a stabilizer. Significant research has been devoted to using it as a renewable resource and as biodiesel for cars.

What Does This Mean For You?

If you have a distended belly, don't overlook fibroids and cysts. There are several reasons why fibroids and cysts occur, but a major cause is excess estrogen and/or hormonal imbalance.

Applying the castor oil packs may help ovarian cysts and fibroids to open and heal. The oil stimulates the area and gets things moving. The oil may also help remove excess estrogen. Sometimes fibroids and cysts go away on their own, and other times they require intervention.

The International Journal of Toxicology[16] reported in a safety assessment that while castor oil was not toxic, they found that ricinoleic acid has a strong suppressive effect on tumors of mice. Ricinoleic fatty acid is the main fat in castor oil.

In a 2009 study[17], scientists studied the effect of castor oil on patients with osteo-arthritis. They administered a capsule of castor oil along with an NSAID (anti-inflammatory drug) pill for four weeks. The patients experienced overall symptom relief after only two weeks of treatment. They reported that the castor oil and NSAID pill was significantly effective against osteo-arthritis.

I use castor oil on my knees in the winter. They tend to ache when I go for walks and run in the cold—especially on rainy days. However, if I apply castor oil beforehand, I can usually bypass the pain. I massage it in to my feet at night too. My feet tend to get achy from all the aerobics I do. Sometimes when I do back-to-back classes, my poor feet can't keep up! All the jumping, stepping, twisting, and turning has my feet on fire by the end of it all. Castor oil gets them soft and pain-free by morning. I just apply it right before I lay down and massage it in for about a minute. They heal overnight.

In another anti-inflammatory study[18], researchers injected carrageenan into the paw of a mouse and histamine into the eyelids of a guinea pig. Poor little guys.

The inflamed thickness was then measured by radioimmunoassay. The purpose of the study was to compare the anti-inflammatory effect of castor oil's ricinoleic acid to capsaicin. Capsaicin is the hot stuff in chili peppers that is already known to have anti-inflammatory effect.

They administered both the castor oil and the capsaicin to the inflamed mouse and guinea pig. After only 8 days of applying both capsaicin and ricinoleic acid (castor oil), the animals showed significant recovery. But the burning effect of capsaicin caused the animals to scratch themselves. They decided to try the ricinoleic acid alone, without the capsaicin. Who needs chili on their eyelids, right?

After trying the ricinoleic acid alone, without the capsaicin, the animals were not irritated. But now they proved that the ricinoleic acid was a much less pungent, yet effective anti-inflammatory.

Interesting that they chose the eyelid. I had a little issue with my own eyelid. I had an attractive sty underneath my right eyelid. You could see a little bump on my eyelid when I closed my eye. It was slightly irritating, but not painful at all.

After 2 weeks with this thing, I decided to soak a cotton ball with some castor oil and place it on my eye while in bed. I left it there for 15-20 minutes, then fell asleep. When I woke up the next day, my eyelid was draining itself! There was little bits of pus coming out of the corner of my eye! At that moment, I was sold. I had just fully removed some crap out of my eye with minimal effort and money. Bonus: no sharp objects were used.

Fluid or pus-filled cysts within the female reproductive system are fairly common. Your body could have already had them, released the pus, and rebuilt its tissue—all without your knowledge.

When the body rebuilds, we are sometimes left with scars, called adhesions. Think of the adhesion like a piece of tape. Your body is trying to heal your open wound, so it will place a piece of tape on your wound over and over again. Sounds great, but this is where the problem begins.

If your body tries to heal itself too quickly, before the cyst is completely empty and clear, the cyst will simply grow and reform under the adhesion. Remember, there's no one down there squeezing the last little bit out as you would do with a pimple. Sometimes the body begins taping itself when the pus is still there. After a while, you have two issues to deal with— the cyst, and the layers of adhesions over the cyst. Some women have pelvises full of fibroids/cysts and adhesions.

Web MD has a comprehensive Visual Guide to Uterine Fibroids[19], where you can see pictures and get more information about fibroids. Remember, getting a diagnosis from the doctor will help you know whether you have them, and which kind you have.

Cayce specifically recommended castor oil for fibroids treatment. The castor oil targets the pelvic region and increases circulation. The oil helps to open and release cysts and reduces inflammation.

So you see, the distended belly that you are obsessed with may not be from eating too much food. It may be from too much junk and inflammation in your pelvic region. When the pus and excessive mucous is removed, and your reproductive system nourished, your belly flattens.

Here's What You'll Need:

1. **1 bottle cold-pressed castor oil.** This can be found at the health food store, or online.
2. **1 large piece of flannel to cover your abdomen.** White is preferred. Do not use any overly colorful flannel, as the dye may penetrate. You can either cut up an

old flannel shirt, or buy chemical-free organic cloths online.

3. **1 electric heating pad.** You can buy this at any drug store.
4. **1 plastic grocery store bag**
5. **1-2 heavy books**

Instructions:

1. A couple hours before bedtime, pour some of the castor oil out onto flannel. Make sure it is soaked.
2. Place the flannel over your belly, covering your lower right ribs (liver), all the way down to your pelvic region.
3. Place the plastic grocery store bag over the flannel to protect the electric heating pad.
4. Turn heating pad to highest setting and place over flannel. Cover belly, liver, and pelvic region with heating pad.
5. Place heavy book over heating pad.
6. Leave treatment on belly 1 to 1.5 hours.

Repeat the procedure for 3 nights. Feel free to use the castor oil pack once or twice per month.

Side Effects and Precautions

Nearly everyone can use castor oil packs, as they are non-toxic and generally regarded as safe. However, if you experience any nausea, diarrhea, dizziness, or shortness of breath, you should discontinue use.

Do not ever ever ever eat the beans, or try to grow and press the oil yourself. This could kill you. Buy the oil already pressed from one of the many natural health food/supplement companies.

Castor oil has been known to induce labor and bring danger to baby. Never use if you are pregnant.

Do not use castor oil if you are diagnosed with appendicitis.

Consuming Castor Oil

Most people find drinking castor oil to be pretty gross, but benefits outweigh bad taste. The oil can be consumed as an occasional laxative, as it does an excellent job of cleansing the entire colon.

There are many good cleanse products on the market today, but castor oil is one of the cheapest, safest methods to cleanse the digestive tract of toxins and parasites.

It is also very simple to have a bottle of castor oil on the shelf, as opposed to various bottles of supplements. From the 1920's through the 1950's, castor oil was a standard substance to have on the shelf, and it was used and even given to children as a way of staying clean.

Unfortunately, many people in Western countries are now under the impression that parasites only exist in underdeveloped countries. After all, we douse ourselves with anti-bacterial products all day, so we should be clean, right?

Our processed food consumption has increased significantly, yet our cleansing has decreased. Many people are not ready to accept that they could have parasites. However, it is estimated that 90% of Americans are hosting parasites within their bodies. Parasites not only leach nutrition from you, they can also eat their way through your organs.

Castor oil and other colon cleansing products are sneaking back onto shelves and becoming more common again. You can find them at regular supermarkets these days. But you should purchase from a trusted health supplement supplier. Buy it online if you don't live near a good health food store.

Laxative and Colon Cleanse

Please note that some castor oil experts argue that ingesting the oil is unnecessary, as the castor oil packs penetrate well enough through the belly. If you still want to try castor oil as a strong laxative, try it first thing in the morning when you are constipated or feel the need to cleanse. Get the okay from your doctor beforehand, of course.

Be sure to limit this cleanse to an occasional thing. If you form a habit out of any laxative, your body can forget how to go to the bathroom on its own. Cleanse once per month, at the most. Remember, do not use castor oil if you are pregnant, as it is known to cause dangerous conditions for the baby.

Here's What You'll Need:

1 ½ -2 oz. cold-pressed castor oil
1 ½ -2 oz. orange juice
Hot water to sip
Lemon and honey

Here's What to Do:

1. Pour castor oil and orange juice in a glass. Hold your nose and chuck it.

2. 15 minutes later, start sipping hot tea, made of hot water, a squeeze of lemon and a teaspoon of honey. Sip three or four cups of this lemon tea.

3. The castor oil will begin flushing your system within a couple hours, depending on how sluggish your digestive system is. Generally, you will go to the bathroom for each cup of hot lemon tea you drink.

When you want to stop flushing, simply introduce a light, healthy meal and stop drinking the tea. A healthy meal could be an apple, and some rice and lentils. Do not consume any fried or processed restaurant meals on this day. Do not consume meat. Keep your meals simple, light, and vegetarian. It is important that you not eat anything crazy when there is nothing in your system. Have you ever not eaten the whole day, and then had some fried chicken? Uggh…stomach pain—or so I've heard. I've never done such a thing, of course.

Another notorious gagger is eating candy or chocolate first thing in the morning.

You might get this feeling if you rush back to eating too soon after a colon cleanse. Your body should be treated delicately after cleansing, reintroducing foods little by little—or else!

Parasite Killer Only

If you only want to kill parasites, and already have regular bowel movements, there is a fairly easy non-gagging way to consume castor oil. It involves using frozen castor oil capsules instead of the free-form liquid in a bottle.

When castor oil is taken in frozen capsule form, the capsules reach all the way to the ileum before they defrost and open. The ileum is located in the last three-fifths of the small intestine, where it's warm and damp—a wonderland for parasites. It will be a giant massacre to any parasites residing here. Yet you never have to smell the oil. Castor oil taken in this form will not cause a laxative effect, but will assist in cleaning the ileum and cecum area where the capsule dissolves.

Chapter Summary

1. Castor oil is scientifically proven to have a positive effect on the lymphatic system.

2. Use the castor oil packs to release trapped mucous and toxins in the belly.

3. Castor oil is an affordable colon cleanser which can relieve constipation.

Chapter Three

Belly-Trimming Fats for Foodies

Coconut Oil's Superiority

One of the best oils you can give your body is coconut oil. This oil will beautify your appearance from the inside out. Thousands of women are using the oil topically to soften and add shine to hair, and to give skin a radiant appearance. One way to take advantage of this oil is to consume it as well. This beneficial oil will even go to work on your brain for you.

Coconut oil easily converts to instant energy. So much so, that the oil is currently being researched as an alternative energy source for the brain. Even Alzheimer's patients are finding relief from coconut oil, since the coconut can provide energy to the brain where patients are lacking a fuel source (glucose).

Coconut oil is broken down by lipase enzymes in saliva, not by the liver. Because the liver and gallbladder are not engaged, they are given time to rest and heal. In addition, the body receives nutrients faster.

Regular consumption of the oil helps to increase metabolism by improving your metabolic rate. According to a 1986 research study published in the American Journal of Clinical Nutrition[20], coconut oil burns fat 3 times faster than other oils.

The oil also slows down absorption of sugar into the bloodstream. It can be very useful for diabetics. It helps reverse insulin resistance by helping the pancreas secrete insulin, according to Dr. Bruce Fife, author of The Coconut Oil Miracle[22].

Coconut oil is a saturated fat, but it is a unique saturated fat. Saturated fats have had a bad reputation for clogging the arteries. Some of the conventional, unnatural saturated fats do. However, coconut oil has been shown to have the opposite effect on the entire cardiovascular system. Many scientists have come to the conclusion that not all saturated fats are created equal. Coconut oil is one of the only oils to contain Medium Chain Fatty Acids. Its coconut oil's Medium Chain Fatty Acids (MCFA's) that make the oil so healthy for your body.

In addition to being used by the brain as an energy source, MCFA's help normalize cholesterol levels by helping to balance the ratio of LDL ("bad" cholesterol) and HDL ("good" cholesterol) in the blood. The lauric acid in coconut oil specifically helps increase good cholesterol. Lauric acid makes monolaurin, a natural antibiotic. Lauric acid is an important ingredient in mothers' breast milk. It's what protects babies from pathogens. Lauric acid and Monolaurin are used to help build the immune system in persons with AIDS. It can also cut down yeast like Candida Albicans.

Coconut is primarily made of the following fatty acids:

Caprylic Acid   9%
Capric Acid   10%
Lauric Acid   52%
Myristic Acid   19%
Palmitic Acid   11%
Oleic Acid   8%
Other/Unknown   5%

Like castor oil, coconut oil improves circulation too. Coconut oil is anti-fungal, anti-parasitic, anti-bacterial, and anti-viral. The oil makes a great cooking oil because its smoking point is high for a healthy cold-pressed oil. As a rule of thumb, use extra-virgin coconut oil if stir-frying or boiling and use refined coconut oil or avocado oil for frying or baking above 350 degrees Fahrenheit. Many raw recipes use coconut oil because it is firm when kept under 75 degrees Fahrenheit.

Most people delight in the smell of coconut oil. But if you are making a dish that doesn't exactly call for the coconutty scent, don't fret; the coconut scent retreats after you add salt.

How Much to Consume

To receive the healthy benefits of coconut oil, you will need to consume 2-3 tablespoons daily. If you tend to avoid eating that much oil because you're always on some kind of low-fat diet, then this will be a real treat for you. Remember the first chapter—like dissolves like. Well, you can lose weight by adding this baby to your diet. So open up and spoon it in.

If you're still having trouble getting it in, try adding a tablespoon to your morning kale shake. It's also delicious on bread, but you didn't read that here.

How to Get it In:

- ✓ 1 tablespoon in a kale shake
- ✓ Spread on bread
- ✓ Cooking oil for stir-frys, soups, and stews
- ✓ As a firming agent for raw desserts
- ✓ Anywhere you can think of under 350 degrees Fahrenheit

What Else Can You Do with Coconut Oil?

Don't forget to massage it into your feet and body. I personally do not use coconut oil near my face or upper arms, because it makes my face break out. Some people naturally have a reaction to the size of coconut oil molecules. They fit perfectly into pores to clog the heck out of them. It doesn't stop me from buying jars and jars of the stuff. I just don't put it anywhere near my face. Everybody is different. That is why you see scores of people recommending it for beautiful soft skin, and other people complaining of acne. See what works for you. Just because your face can't handle it doesn't mean your hands won't look young and beautiful from daily use. You can always find use for coconut oil. It's a good lubricant for sex too.

Olive Oil

No health book would be complete without mention of olive oil. Olive oil is the queen of oils, because people all over the world have been using it for centuries. And the oil still stands up. It is not faddish, like canola oil (more on this in Chapter 5). There is no trend with olive oil. It is simply time-tested and true.

It can be less expensive than some of the other healthy oils, and it is available everywhere. When you purchase your extra-virgin olive oil, make sure it is packaged in a dark amber, glass container. Do not go for the Costco-sized mega-containers unless they are dark. Even so, if you are going Costco-sized, just remember that oils have an expiration date, and the longer an oil sits on the shelf, the less potent it will be. If you buy a big vat of olive oil, make sure you can use it. Of all oils, olive oil has the most selection at the supermarket. Some markets go crazy with their selection of olive oils. Remember the following when choosing an oil:

Nutrients are preserved in the oil of dark glass bottles. Generally speaking, the better packaged an oil, the more the manufacturer cared about the product inside. Who would tend to the finest olives, take care harvesting the olives, use special extraction methods to avoid harming the olives, and then pack it all up in the cheapest plastic they can find? Dark glass is the easiest way to ensure you are getting a fine oil from a good manufacturer. Plastic is okay, but glass always trumps plastic.

UV and heat destroy both plastic and oil. Some oils have a tendency of having a very short shelf life. It is not a bad tendency. Actually, the more perishable an oil is, the healthier it is for you. But you don't want an oil that is so perishable that it is rancid by the time you use it. Olive oil can sit on a shelf for a couple of years without going rancid. Sure, the nutrition will be reduced each month, but the oil will not become completely rancid unless you completely lose your head for two years and forget that it is there. You also have no idea how long an oil has been sitting on a supermarket shelf unless the bottle contains both the stamped manufacture date and the expiration date. Consuming rancid oils can increase your risk for cancer, as oils become carcinogenic.

Avoid purchasing oils from aluminum tin cans. Metal tends to destroy oils over time, and the soldering used to seal can parts together may contain lead.

Choose a manufacturer who appears to care about your oil. Olive oil is like fine wine. You want an oil connoisseur to hand you that bottle of oil, not the company that just figured out how to slash prices, thus slashing quality. Some olive oils can be laden with chemicals, as olives can be high in pesticides. You can avoid chemicals by either choosing organic, or choosing a manufacturer who cares about the product so much that he would never dream of ruining his product with a load of ill-flavored chemicals.

When you get home, don't store olive oils near the stove or out on the counter. Store them inside your cabinet, in a sealed container. If you are wondering about the cabinet above the stove, check it. If it is cool, it is fine to store oils there. When you use the oil, replace the top and put the oil back into the dark, cool cabinet. Extra-virgin olive oil does not need refrigeration like some of the other oils, but do keep it stored dark and cool.

Make sure you buy "extra-virgin" olive oil. "Pure" or "Light" olive oil, or oil with anything other than the words "virgin" attached to it, is not worth consuming. Non-virgin oil has almost always been manipulated by bleaching, deodorizing, de-gumming, refining, etc. Processing oil this way removes all nutrition and is hazardous to your health.

If you remember one thing and one thing only about extra-virgin olive oil, let it be this:

Never fry food with Extra-Virgin Olive Oil

Extra-virgin olive oils should always be kept below 325 degrees Fahrenheit. It is not just a question of losing powerful healing benefits. You will be turning your house into a trans-fat factory if you heat it above this temperature. You will be risking both heart disease and cancer by eating this way. Use extra-virgin coconut oil instead. You can also add oil to your dish after cooking. Making Spaghetti Bolognese? Brown the meat in either its own fat, or a little coconut oil. Then add 1-2 tablespoons of extra-virgin olive oil at the end. Your guests will appreciate the olive oil aroma in the food, and you'll win extra points by not giving them heart disease.

70

It is okay to add extra-virgin olive oil to soups, stews, and beans while they are still cooking because the oil will only get as hot as the boiling temperature. But the moment we fry, bake, broil, and grill foods, the temperature reaches far beyond 232 degrees Fahrenheit. Eating fried and grilled food is bad in itself. You don't want to pour gas on the fire by throwing in some trans-fat too. If you've got to have that olive oil flavor because you need that Italian/Mediterranean taste and feel, just add it afterward when the food is off the fire. The oils in the food will taste better. The food will look moister and more scrumptious too.

If you're from a family like mine, it's a cardinal sin to not brown everything in oil before pouring in water or stock. I just ignore this. I don't want to be unhealthy just so I can hang on to the tradition of browning things. We don't need to fry every little thing we get our hands on. Vegetables lose the health aspect when browned. As soon as you begin browning or scorching a vegetable, consider its molecular structure changed forever. You are now eating an engineered food, inspired by you.

Its fine sometimes. We gotta live, right? But you don't need to religiously fry food before making such things as soups or stews. Save your fry points for when you are dying for french fries or spring rolls. Don't spend your fry points on soup. Soup is better without all the frying anyway. Simply add your ingredients to a little bit of water or stock, and keep adding water as you add ingredients, little by little. Add your oil near the end. Do the same with beans and stews.

You can also try the following method if you want to avoid frying:

Use a small amount of water in the fry-pan, so that you are actually "steaming" the food, not frying. The cooking temperature of steaming is much lower and healthier than frying. It will keep the temperature down to 212 degrees Fahrenheit or 100 degrees Celsius, and you won't be scorching your food. When you are almost done cooking your dish, bring on the glorious oil.

Blame bad cholesterol and clogged arteries on the method of cooking. Not on the healthy oil.

Burning Belly Fat with Extra-Virgin Olive Oil

Olive oil has been studied to be a thermogenic food, which means that it gives your body heat, increasing the basal metabolic rate. This increase in metabolism will also increase your energy expenditure, resulting in fat loss.

A Japanese study[23] on rats concluded that the oil enhanced thermogenesis by increasing the uncoupling protein in brown adipose tissue. Brown adipose tissue is the good type of body fat that helps you burn energy. Newborns have this type of fat, but as we get older, brown adipose tissue decreases. Extra-virgin olive oil stimulates the brown fat you still have, so that you can burn the bad fat known as "white fat." Its good news if you are a rat.

Not only does extra-virgin olive oil stimulate thermogenesis, but it is also known to be anabolic. It can increase muscle mass by stimulating muscle growth. You will definitely need to lift weights to make this work. No single food will increase muscle mass unless you use it along with some strength-building exercise like weight-lifting or yoga.

Studies have also shown that you are less likely to be obese when consuming extra-virgin olive oil because of its tendency to break down fat more than other oils. "Lypolysis," is the process of removing unwanted fatty deposits. It's the lipolytic activity in extra-virgin olive oil which helps break down and release fat within your cells.

Extra-virgin olive oil will also help you feel full longer. A recent study in Germany[24] found that when olive oil was added to participants' morning yogurt for three months, the group did not gain weight, meaning they maintained their weight throughout the study. The scientists observed that hormone serotonin levels were higher in the participants, and that participants felt a sense of increased satiety, or feeling of satisfaction with the meal.

Cleansing with Olive Oil

The olive oil cleanse is a liver and gallbladder cleanse, but your entire bodily system could benefit from this cleanse—clearer skin, more energy, smaller waistline. This cleanse is an adaptation from Dr. Hulda Clarke's Liver Cleanse. Here is a helpful page about the cleanse: Cure Zone[25].

If you are obese, meaning 20 lbs. over your target weight or you are over 20% body fat, you may have already developed gallstones in your gallbladder. Imagine how much better you would look and feel if you physically removed a pound of stones from your abdomen. This cleanse will do much more than that. You want your liver and gallbladder to be free of stones, so that you can properly digest nutrition and discard toxins. Even if you are certain you do not have gallstones, you can still benefit from this cleanse. After all, toxins don't always come in the form of stones, right? If you take care of your liver and gallbladder, your liver and gallbladder will take care of you. And you will have a much easier time slimming your belly.

The gallbladder works in conjunction with the liver. When you eat, your liver produces bile. The gallbladder collects the bile and stores it there. It then releases some to the small intestine to help digest fats. But bile can't handle it all. Not all fat dissolves easily in bile. Some fat, like cholesterol, does not break down easily. When the fat doesn't dissolve, it forms clumps. The clumps can crystalize, and voila—you have your precious stones. Stones can be all different—from a tiny particle of sand, to an uncomfortable 4-centimeter size. You are probably wondering if you have any of these little stones. Here are some of the symptoms:

- No symptoms at all
- Jaundice in very severe cases
- Gas & Bloating
- Inflammation of gallbladder, liver, pancreas, bile ducts in very severe cases

Gallstones are usually detected by ultrasound while a doctor is looking for something else. Twenty percent of the U.S. population have gallstones, so it's fairly common. However, eighty percent of people who have gallstones do not report any symptoms at all. The majority of people who have gallstones have no idea they have them.

Sometimes stones exit through the bile duct on their own, but other times, they hang out in the gallbladder. It is pretty rare for a stone to get caught in the bile duct and clog, but it does happen to 3% of people that have gallstones. The purpose of this cleanse is to get these crystalized stones to painlessly dissolve and exit stage left.

Before performing this cleanse, you should do a parasite cleanse. Yes, there is that ugly word again. But there isn't a lot of use in cleansing, if parasites can just come knock everything over. The point of a cleanse is to rid of all predators and to get your body to function the way it's supposed to. Parasites are destructive, and will sabotage your efforts to have a healthy, functioning body. It's a waste of money and effort not to rid of parasites before any cleanse. In addition, you could feel ill or nauseous after the gallbladder cleanse if you have not completed the parasite cleanse beforehand. Do complete the parasite cleanse directly before the Olive Oil Cleanse.

Many people that perform this cleanse report amazing results, but that doesn't mean you will too. Your body might hate this cleanse. Everyone is different. You should consult with a doctor before performing this cleanse, to ensure that this cleanse is safe and healthy for you.

This cleanse uses magnesium sulfate, also known as Epsom salt to dilate bile ducts and smoothen muscle. It is a laxative that will help speed the elimination of stones during the cleanse. People have died from overdosing on Epsom salt. It's extremely important to make sure your body tolerates Epsom salt before consuming the amount in this cleanse. Do not skip this step. If your digestion is sensitive, use less Epsom salt. If you do not want to use Epsom salt, you can use prune juice. Prune juice will help you eliminate, but will be less strong.

Here's What You'll Need:

- ✓ Extra-virgin olive oil
- ✓ 3 lbs. apples, organic preferred
- ✓ 5 liters unfiltered apple juice, organic preferred. This should be cloudy, not clear.
- ✓ 3 tbs. apple cider vinegar (containing the "mother")
- ✓ Small box Epsom salt (or prune juice—see note above)

✓ Grapefruit juice from 1 freshly squeezed grapefruit. Fresh lemon juice can be substituted.
✓ Salads and light vegetables to eat for 3 days
✓ Drinking straws, optional
✓ Plastic colander, optional
✓ Herbal tea, optional

Here's What to Do:

Begin three days in advance with apples, apple juice, apple cider, and salads. If you currently eat meat, begin limiting both meat and fat on the first two days. On the third day, completely cut out all meat and fat. This is a preparation for the liver. Drink 1-2 liters of apple juice per day, and eat as many apples as you like. The malic acid in apples will help open bile ducts and soften stones. Have 1 tablespoon of the apple cider vinegar along with your apple juice once each day for the first three days. It is fine to go to work on the first three days, but on the fourth and fifth day, you should stay home and rest.

Day 1: Eat: Apples, 1 tablespoon apple cider vinegar, 1-2 liters apple juice, light meals like soups and salads, limit meat and fat/oils

Day 2: Eat: Apples, 1 tablespoon apple cider vinegar, 1-2 liters apple juice, light meals like soups and salads, limit meat and fat/oils

Day 3: Eat: No Meat, no fats, no oils. Apples, 1 tablespoon apple cider vinegar, 1-2 liters apple juice, light meals like soups and salads

The cleanse begins on day 4 in the morning. It is best not to go anywhere for the next couple days because you will be eliminating, resting, and busy following cleanse instructions. You will want to do the cleanse on your days off from work.

Day 4: Big breakfast (see below) and cleanse. Stay home. Eat no meat, no oils, no fats.

Big breakfast: Eat a big no-meat, no-oil breakfast, consisting of foods that will sustain you for the next 24 hours. The meal can consist of grains, fruits, veggies, or soup. Make sure to exclude all oils, fats, and meats.

2 p.m. No more food. Stop eating food altogether. You may drink herbal tea, a small amount of apple juice, and a small amount of lemon and honey mixed in water. Have plenty of fresh plain water.

6 p.m. Take one teaspoon Epsom salt and mix with one cup of apple juice. Drink it as quickly as you need to. Follow with one cup of fresh, plain water.

8 p.m. Do the same procedure as you did at 8 pm-- take one teaspoon Epsom salt and mix with one cup of apple juice. Drink it as quickly as you need to. Follow with one cup of fresh, plain water.

9:30 p.m. Get ready for bed. You will need to go to bed immediately after the next step, so you'll want to do whatever bedtime chores you have now.

10 p.m. Take olive oil-grapefruit juice mixture. Take a ½ cup olive oil and mix with a ½ cup grapefruit juice in a jar and shake to mix. Drink as quickly as you like. You may feel nauseated at this point. Drinking from a straw can help. Brush your teeth, go potty, then go to bed immediately. In bed, lie on your right side in the fetal position. It's fine to switch to your favorite position during the night, but begin in this position and stay in this position as long as possible.

Day 5—Elimination Day. Its action time.

7 a.m. Take 2 teaspoons Epsom salt (yes, one more spoon than yesterday) mixed with 1 cup apple juice. Go back to bed or enjoy a book or television. You will have bowel movements a little later, in the late morning/early afternoon.

10 am. Decide whether to take 2 more teaspoons Epsom salt mixed with 1 cup apple juice. If you have good bowel movements already, there's probably no need to take. If you haven't had a bowel movement yet, consider taking.

Afternoon- You can eat light meals after you have had 2-3 bowel movements on this day. Do not consume any meat until the following day. Stick to soups, salads, juice, and water.

It can be fun to collect your stones to see your success. If you would like to do this, use a plastic colander to catch the stones as you have your bowel movements. Then pour a picture of hot water over the stones and into the toilet.

Good job! Have a blast collecting your stones. Victory!

Lovely Oily Foods

If the thought of consuming fresh oils makes you want to gag, you're in luck. There's a few foods you can indulge in all month long. Consider splurging on the Olive Oil Cleanse once or twice a year, but consume good oily foods year-round, on the regular basis.

One of the best beauty foods is avocado. These little guys are well-worth your money and effort because they are power-packed with the kind of beauty and nutrition that every woman wants.

The oil in avocado is monounsaturated fat, like extra-virgin olive oil. Avocados also contain fiber, phytochemicals, and numerous vitamins and minerals. In 2013, data[44] was collected from 17,567 people between the ages of 19 and 50. Only 2% of people were regular consumers of avocado. They found that waist circumference, Body Mass Index (BMI), and weight were significantly lower in the individuals who consumed avocados. They also concluded that people who consumed avocados had better dietary intake, better nutrient quality, and a reduced risk of metabolic syndrome.

One out of six people in the U.S. have metabolic syndrome, according to the American Heart Association. It is not really a single disease, but more like a vicious circle, also known as "Syndrome X." It is a group of symptoms including high blood pressure, high blood sugar, high bad cholesterol level, and too much abdominal fat. Syndrome X then leads you to the actual disease—heart attack, stroke, diabetes. It's not pretty. According to the American Heart Association and the National Heart, Lung, and Blood Institute, if you have any 3 of the following symptoms, you are probably in Syndrome X:

> Large Waist Size: Men: 40 inches or larger is too much. Women: 35 inches or larger is too much

> Cholesterol: LDL (Bad): Both Sexes: Either 160 mg/dL or higher OR taking cholesterol pills

> Cholesterol: HDL (Good): Men: less than 40 mg/dL OR taking cholesterol pills. Women: less than 50 mg/dL OR taking cholesterol pills

> High Blood Pressure: Either having blood pressure measuring 135/85 mm Hg or more OR taking blood pressure pills

> ➢ Blood Sugar: High Fasting Glucose Level: 100 mg/dL or higher

An avocado is not the cure for being fat or having heart disease. There's no magic pill, but with enough changes, anything can be reversed. Activity and food are principle to staying healthy. Most people already know they should be working out, so there's not much reason to bash anyone over the head with a barbell. You gotta workout—walk, run, join aerobics classes, practice yoga. This book is to help you with the little problem areas that won't go away, like your little kangaroo pouch.

Out of a 322-calorie avocado, a whopping 44% of it is fat. 21% is saturated and the rest is mono and polyunsaturated fat. How could avocado-eaters be so skinny, chowing down on something so fattening? Doesn't this totally mess up what we grew up believing about fat? We learned to lay off the guacamole and go for the "light" sour cream when eating tacos. But we need that avocado to battle the bulge.

Avocados contain the same monounsaturated fatty acid as extra-virgin olive oil: oleic fatty acid. The oleic fatty acid improves insulin insensitivity, induces fat burning, and helps to reduce appetite.

The omega-3 fatty acid, alpha-Linolenic acid, ALA is also present in avocados. It has been shown to enhance the effects of fat-loss by improving metabolism and cholesterol.

The avocado itself, is fully loaded with phytosterols and carotenoids. It's the wide variety of carotenoids that gives it its anti-inflammatory properties.

Go Nuts

Nuts are tricky. Consuming them is an absolute must, but overdo it and you're screwed. These babies are densely packed with nutrition and good fat. They also contain a small amount of protein, so you can use them as a quick snack to get you to your next meal. But nuts have more fat than protein, so trying to use them as a protein source might just get you fat instead.

They also contain fiber and minerals. The best beauty nuts tend to be almonds, walnuts, and Brazil nuts, but all nuts can be helpful towards improving your nutrition and helping you lose weight, provided you do not eat too many.

Peanuts mold very quickly, so it is advisable not to eat many of these, or go too crack-addict on the peanut butter, as you do not need any extra mold growing in your belly. While some people are deathly allergic to peanuts, many others have an ongoing peanut intolerance and don't even know it.

Pistachios also have a little mold problem, where the hulls can break open before they are harvested, leaving the food inside susceptible to mold and bacteria. Breaking these open and popping them in your mouth is addictive. If you know you can't stop, buy them for special occasions only.

Always try to go raw when choosing nuts. This will minimize your trans-fat intake, and you will get the most bang for your buck. Roasted nuts usually contain a lot of sodium. Even if you get "low-sodium" nuts, you are still eating the bad oil they poured on to roast the nuts, and then you are getting an alteration of the good oil. Any heat alteration of a good oil, makes it a not-so-good oil. Run for the hills if you see nuts labeled "sweet."

It is important to note that the jury is still out on whether nuts help you lose weight. But they can and should be used in conjunction with a fat-loss program because they provide a natural way to ward off hunger, they are a quick nutrient-dense snack, and they contain beautifying fats that help you stay young and healthy.

Some scientific evidence does point toward weight loss. In an article in The American Journal of Clinical Nutrition[26], Joan Sabaté pointed out that people who ate nuts excreted more fat in their stools. Another study[27] showed that people who ate nuts were less likely to be obese, meaning that weight gain was less common. While further research needs to be completed on whether nuts help you lose weight, you can still enjoy nuts knowing that you are getting healthier.

Go Fish

One of the most amazing beauty foods on the planet are fish like salmon, mackerel, herring, sardines and fish roe. If you want to get your omega-3 from a natural food source with minimal supplementation, this is a good way. These cold-water fish come heavily loaded with omega-3 in the form of both DHA and EPA. You'll read more about DHA and EPA in the next chapter. For now, just know that they are essential, meaning your body can not make them on its own—kind of like our essential amino acids and our need for protein. You gotta have it if you want to be healthy. You want to aim for 2000-3000 milligrams of omega-3 fatty acids per day.

The question is, how much salmon can you handle per week without becoming violently ill from mercury poisoning? A 3-oz serving of salmon will give you 1000-1500 milligrams omega-3. Include this in your diet two to three times per week. This means you can skip fish oil pills on the days you eat salmon, or another omega-3 loaded fish. If you choose salmon, make sure you eat Alaskan wild salmon which will minimize your exposure to toxins like mercury and PCB's (Polychlorinated Biphenyls).

The other fish that are heavily-loaded with EPA and DHA are mackerel (avoid King Mackerel which contains too much toxins and too little omega-3), sardines, herring, anchovies, Greenland halibut, and Pacific Northwest oysters. Oh...and fish roe.

What's fish roe? Fish eggs! Sounds disgusting, but they're actually quite tasty, and quite common in many parts of the world.

The fish roe that packs the most power to the punch when it comes to omega-3 is caviar, weighing in at 5000 grams of DHA and EPA per 3 ounces. Only problem is, caviar is taken from endangered fish. Beluga, from the Sturgeon family is highly endangered. As a matter of fact, nearly all Sturgeon are endangered, so we should even avoid imitation caviar. Imitation caviar is most often times made from other fish in the Sturgeon family. Both true and imitation caviar is black in color. Caviar is not on the chart below, because we're not getting that. It's simply too endangered.

However, you don't need to avoid roe entirely. The reddish-orange variety that you might find as a sushi garnishment is salmon roe. You can also find roe from cod, lumpfish, sea urchin, and many more types of fish. It's pretty affordable and convenient. You can find it in both cans and plastic containers in ethnic markets or ethnic sections of grocery stores.

All cans and types of preparation are fine, when it comes to omega-3 fish. Watch for fish canned in oil though. This can raise your omega-6 level, unless it is canned in extra-virgin olive oil. Also remember that the higher the temperature, the more damaged the molecules will be. Frying fish will undermine your efforts to get your omega-3. Opt for baking or steaming. Or straight out of the can.

Check out the following chart to see how different foods stack up next to each other. This will help you determine how much you need of each food to get the right amount of EPA and DHA. Remember, you are shooting for 2000-3000 mg (2-3 grams) daily. Your best bet is supplementation, along with eating some of the high DHA/EPA foods. ALA, omega-6, total fat, and protein is compared on the chart as well.

Comprehensive Omega-3/Omega-6 Chart

			EPA (mg)	DHA (mg)	ALA (mg)	Omega-3 (mg)	Omega-6 (mg)	Fat Total (g)	Protein (g)
Atlantic Farmed Salmon, 3 oz.			587	1238	96	1921	566	10.5	19
Alaska Salmon, Chinook, 3 oz.			859	618	94	1822	116	11	22
Alaska Salmon Coho, 3 oz.			462	706	169	1587	221	6	23
Alaska Salmon Sockeye, 3 oz.			450	595	53	1210	96	9	

Herring, 3 oz.		773	939	112	1885	142	10	20
Mackerel, Jack, Canned, 3 oz.		369	675	36	1167	84	5.4	21
Mackerel, Pacific & Jack, 3 oz.		555	1016	54	1759	127	9	22
Fish Roe, 3 oz.		1071	1485	6.8	2651	31.5	7	24
Pacific Oysters, steamed, 3 oz.		745	425	54	1258	54	4	16
Sardines, canned in tomato sauce, 3 oz.		447	726	197	1422	103	9	18
Anchovies, canned drained, 3 oz.		648	1095	14.4	1791	306	9	24
Pastured Pork, 3 oz.		Unknown/ Not enough info						
Pastured Beef, Ground, 3 oz.		1	0	20	74	360	12	15
Past. Beef,		2	0	13	18	67	2	18

Steak, 3 oz.							
Pastured Chicken 3 oz.	0	0	0.02	0.1	0.6	3	26
Pastured Eggs, 2, 3 oz.	0	0	1.3	1.3	Unknown	10	12
Regular Lard, 1 Tbs.	0	0	128	128	1300	13	0
Pastured Lard, 1 Tbs.	Unknown/Not Enough info						
Regular Beef Tallow, 1 Tbs.	0	0	76.5	76.5	395	13	0
Pastured Beef Tallow, 1 Tbs.	0	0	104	104	143	13	0
Regular Butter	0	0	44.1	44.1	382	11	0
Pastured Butter	9	1.31		Unknown/Not enough info		11	0
Goose Fat, , 1 T	0	0	53.8	53.8	1250	13	0

The American Heart Association recommends not to eat more than two 3-oz servings, but many people in other cultures eat fish every day, or every other day. It could be that the other components of their diet allow them to handle heavy metals. For instance, a diet with lots of cilantro or rau ram helps detoxify the body of mercury on the regular basis.

On the other hand, maybe they shouldn't be eating fish every day and just haven't caught up with the new guidelines. Who knows? Our seawaters get more and more contaminated as years pass. Things change. It is sad to think that there could come a time when we can't enjoy wild fish at all without risking mercury and/or PCB poisoning. Fortunately, the United Nations has put together a mercury convention, known as The Minamata Convention on Mercury, committed to protecting both humans and the environment.

You should definitely watch your intake if you are pregnant or nursing. If you have concerns about eating fish, take omega-3 in supplement form only. Most brands have very low Mercury, or Mercury-free and PCB-free.

The beautiful part about eating omega-3-rich fish is that you are also getting lean protein, vitamin D, selenium, zinc, and B vitamins. It's ridiculously nutritious. But it has drawbacks—fish oil pills are regarded by many as unsustainable for the environment, and a not-so-nice way to treat fish.

If you want to avoid fish altogether, reach for the algae pills. There is a reason why fish have so much omega-3 after all. Eat what the fish eats. Well, salmon are omnivores, but they do feed on sea plants, and prey on other fish which feed on algae.

Chapter Summary

1. Never fry food using extra-virgin olive oil. Use coconut oil instead.

2. Buy quality extra-virgin olive oil in dark glass bottles.

3. Coconut, avocado, and olive oil improve metabolism and help cut belly fat.

Chapter Four

Shiny Oil Supplements

Supplementation is the best way to meet omega-3 daily requirements. While coconut oil, olive oil, and castor oil are optional, omega-3 oils are essential. They are an absolute must for health. Not only do our bodies thrive on fatty acids, but we become ill if we do not have enough. We have many "essential" nutrients that our bodies require, yet cannot make on our own. We have all of our essential amino acids, our essential vitamins and minerals, and we have our essential fats.

The two essential fatty acids are polyunsaturated fats, called omega-3 and omega-6. In this chapter we will look at these fatty acids, how to get them in. We will also sort out what to do if you follow a vegan diet. Lastly, we will look at perhaps one of the most interesting and unusual ways to supplement with oil—oil pulling.

In a research study published in 2010 in the American Journal of Clinical Nutrition[28], scientists examined the ongoing problem of losing muscle mass with age. The condition, called sarcopenia affects nearly everyone, but it especially affects those who do not exercise. They looked to omega-3 for the answer. They gave sixteen, healthy older adults a supply of either corn oil or omega-3 oil. After 8 weeks, they found that while corn oil did nothing, the omega-3 fatty acids stimulated muscle protein synthesis. Corn oil is fairly high in omega-6 fatty acids.

Omega-6 oils are essential, and they are not all bad. One of the main problems is that we get way too much of them. They include corn oil, sunflower oil, sesame oil, and soybean oil. They are also sold under the blanket term, "vegetable oil."

Coconut oil is neither an omega-3 oil, nor an omega-6 oil, although it does contain a trivial amount of omega-6.

Ratio is key to understanding the omegas and how much to get of each. For every one omega-6 fat, you should get one omega-3 fat. The Standard American diet is currently at about 10-20 to 1, meaning that for every 10-20 omega-6 servings, you then squeeze in one measly serving of omega-3. The lack of omega-3 could be the reason why our cancer and cardiovascular disease rates are so high.

Omega-6 oils are completely necessary for the body and are responsible for creating an inflammatory environment for your body. If you sprain your ankle, omega-6 steps in and says, "Hey ya'll, inflame that so that she knows something ain't right! Fire it up!"

It's a very useful signal that can help prevent serious illness by causing awareness. Some people battle inflammation all their lives, and it never advances to a more serious level. Monitoring and keeping inflammation at bay is an ongoing goal and lifestyle for many people. If you keep inflammation at bay in a healthy manner—naturally—it means you're winning. If you keep inflammation at bay with a daily dose of drugs like Advil or Aleve, you are cheating. Furthermore, it is unclear whether you are actually winning or losing. NSAID drugs come with a whole slew of problems, from an overworked liver to toxic kidneys. Sure, you get rid of the pain, but the consequences of not solving the underlying issue could be severe.

Any disease containing the ending "-itis," usually refers to inflammation. Laryngitis is inflammation of the larynx. Appendicitis is inflammation of the appendix. Arthritis is inflammation of the joints. Many Western doctors advocate removing the inflamed part. If a child's tonsils cause too much trouble, take 'em out.

Indeed, sometimes removal of a part can mean life or death, especially with something like appendicitis. But it is sometimes best to examine why the inflame response got signaled in the first place. We must also remember that if we are missing one of those the next time the area gets inflamed, we will have a tougher time figuring out what is wrong.

Tendinitis, arthritis, and gingivitis are all inflammatory responses to an underlying issue. Wouldn't it be nice if we had an anti-inflammatory response as well? We can have that! That's where omega-3 comes in. Omega-3 creates an anti-inflammatory response within the body. Any inflammatory issue can be improved and healed with omega-3 oils.

Omega-3 itself does not heal any disease. Omega-3 oils improve the structure of your cells so that cells can do their jobs within your body. We all have bad cells, or cells that are not doing their job at any given point. These are cancerous cells. It is only a problem when many, many cells in the same area begin to fail at their job. This is cancer. All disease is the consequence of unhealthy cells. Omega-3 tries to get all cells, everywhere in the body, to a functional state.

There are 3 main types of essential omega-3 fatty acids:

> ALA (alpha-Linolenic acid) is a polyunsaturated fat, with 18 carbons and 3 double bonds. Found abundantly in: flax, hemp, chia, lingonberry, kiwi seeds and walnuts. It is a shorter-chained, simple omega-3. We cannot make ALA from scratch. Theoretically, you can ingest ALA and then your body can convert it to EPA, and later to DHA. But

this has an efficiency rate of 5%. It converts pretty poorly. If you are relying on ALA to get cover your omega-3 requirement, you need another method unless you are hardcore raw vegan. Read on.

➢ EPA (Eicosapentaenoic Acid) is a polyunsaturated fat with 20 carbons and 5 double bonds. Found abundantly in: Fish, shellfish, algae, krill. EPA is a precursor to DHA. When you purchase an omega-3 supplement, or eat fish, you are usually getting a combination of EPA and DHA. You rarely find one without the other. We cannot make EPA from scratch. It must be consumed or converted from ALA or we will face deficiencies that lead to illness.

➢ DHA (Docosahexaenoic acid) is a polyunsaturated fat with 22 carbons and 6 double bonds. Found abundantly in: Fish, shellfish, algae, krill. DHA is the primary component of the brain, skin and retina. DHA has been shown to inhibit cancer cell growth, and improve mental and cardiovascular health. It has also been studied to help burn fat and build muscle. Mothers pass DHA to babies through breastfeeding, as breast milk is high in DHA. We cannot make DHA from scratch. It must be consumed or converted from ALA and EPA or we will face deficiencies that lead to illness.

It's the double bond in the omega-3's that make them more flexible and interactive with cells, but it is also what makes the oil susceptible to damage through light and heat. Each cell is surrounded by a fat membrane. A rigid, yet flexible fat membrane will cause a cell to function well.

All cells work together in a complex system. One of a cell's jobs is to send and receive messages from and to the other cells. They combine together to build muscle and skin tissue—yes, that means muscle tone and better skin if you have optimum cell performance. If the fat membrane of a cell is too rigid, it will not be able to communicate with the other cells.

Omega-3 helps a cell become more permeable by improving the fluidity of the membrane. The membrane becomes more flexible, and your system flows better. Nutrients are passed through the cell membrane into the cell, and waste products are passed out of the cell through the cell membrane. And you know what happens when a cell can remove waste properly. You remove fat properly.

EPA and DHA doesn't only touch the membrane of the cell, it improves the functionality of the nucleus and mitochondrion inside the cell. The nucleus contains information that helps the cell reproduce to make more cells. This is a strong key point to anyone who is aging. Wait, that's everyone.

Cells die every day. Each day, adults will lose roughly 50-70 billion cells per day, but the good news is that more cells are being reproduced to replace those that died. However, as we age, the ovaries, the kidneys, the liver, and the brain slow down in cell production. Any disorder or illness may also result in a drop in new cell production.

This is also why you see that horrid decrease in muscle tone, beginning at the age of 30. Muscle cells will be slashed if you don't work out. Use it or lose it. Muscle loss becomes very evident in older people that don't exercise. They could get away with it in their youth, but all that inactivity will show as they start losing muscle cells and muscle growth. Luckily, it's possibly to turn it around with some strength exercises.

Amazingly, cells have been studied to have a programmed death in a normal health situation. But then there's the free radicals. Sounds like a cool hippie band, but it's not. When the free radicals come around, they do damage to cells, which will cause premature cell death.

Rice University in Houston[29] defined free radicals as, "atoms or groups of atoms with an odd (unpaired) number of electrons and can be formed when oxygen interacts with certain molecules. Once formed, these highly reactive radicals can start a chain reaction, like dominoes. Their chief danger comes from the damage they can do when they react with important cellular components such as DNA, or the cell membrane. Cells may function poorly or die if this occurs. " The article then goes on to explain that anti-oxidants are used by the body to interact and terminate free radicals' chain reaction event and that anti-oxidants must come from the diet.

Remember, EPA and DHA will help protect the membrane as well, so eat a diet rich in fruits and vegetables, and then add in the omega-3 supplement.

Then there is the mitochondrion inside a cell which helps make energy by using oxygen to break down food. That's why a breath of fresh air will help you think better, help you lift something heavy, and help you de-stress—it's the oxygen you need...and well-functioning cells. And of course, good food.

In a 2010 European study[30], 25 obese adolescents were given 1.2 grams per day of omega-3 fatty acids, or a placebo for three months. Researchers found improved vascular health in the teens that took the omega-3. They also noted a decline in inflammation in the obese teens.

The idea is to get omega-3 to help your cells out as much as they can, so that they can reproduce, take in good nutrients for your body, and dispose of waste and toxins. DHA and EPA have the following benefits when it comes to fat loss and muscle building:

Increases muscle anabolism: This happens when the body takes substances and uses them to build muscle tissue. Athletes who risked their lives using steroids could have used omega-3 and a few other essentials instead. Anabolism is the opposite of catabolism. Catabolism is where the body breaks down and loses tissue because it is starved for nutrition.

Preserve existing muscle gain: Omega-3 serves to protect all cells, including muscle cells. Taking a good source of omega-3 will make a cell better able to ward off free radical damage.

Reduces inflammation: Get those muscles and joints working better with some lube. Omega-3 is a powerful anti-inflammatory that will decrease muscle soreness.

Vegans and Vegetarians: Eat What the Fish Ate

If you are trying to get your omega-3 from flaxseed oil, hempseed oil, or chia seeds, it may not work very well. Indeed, these seeds contain ALA, the primary building block for DHA. But it's actually the DHA that you need, and you can achieve that easier through just supplementing with DHA. Theoretically, if you are on a strict raw vegan diet where you eat no junk food, and have no digestive issues, you should be able to convert ALA to DHA in about 10 months from the time you begin. If you are on the raw diet, be sure to make a lot of your meals with the good oils—and use them liberally. Good

ALA oils come from hemp, flax, and chia. A raw vegan may be able to make enough DHA if their diet is stellar.

However, most people that need omega-3 have digestive issues and most people that have digestive issues need omega-3. And if you've got a belly, you've got digestive issues. Our bodies have a very poor conversion rate from ALA to DHA. We have a hard time metabolizing ALA. A fish has a much easier time converting the algae and phytoplankton to DHA and EPA. Then it retains its fat because of the cold temperature. We need to supplement in order to get DHA.

So what can you do if you're vegan? Eat what the fish ate. Load up on algae. And when supplementing with the flax, hemp, and chia, eat them with the following vitamins and minerals to enhance conversion:

1. Vitamin C
2. Vitamins B6 & B12
3. Zinc
4. Magnesium

Taking these supplements along with the seeds will give your body a better chance at converting the seed oils into DHA. If you are following the vegan diet well, and not eating vegan mac & cheese for dinner, then you are probably already getting enough nutrients. You can always have a metabolic panel done at your doctor's office to see what your deficiencies are. If you don't have insurance, cough up some cash and have one done. That way you can make an informed decision. If you are depressed and vegan, use the algae oil.

Just because hemp, flax, and chia only provide ALA (not DHA/EPA), it doesn't mean they're off-limits. They are still beautiful seed oils and should still be consumed to your heart's content. There is some question about whether flax is too phytoestrogenic (a food that mimics estrogen in the body), but it probably is not nearly as problematic as the phytoestrogen king--soy. It's probably fine to ingest a couple tablespoons of these omega-rich seeds once a day. If you are at all weary about the possibility of messing with your hormones, just buy hemp or chia. Here is how the seeds and oils stack up to one another:

1 tablespoon Chia Seeds:
Fiber................5 g
Protein............2.5g
EPA & DHA.......0
ALA............... 2400 mg
Omega-6............800 mg
Price............$ .22

1 tablespoon Hemp Seeds:
Fiber.............. .3 g
Protein............3.5g
EPA & DHA.......0
ALA............... 1000 mg
Omega-6..........2500 mg
Price......... ....$ .26

1 tablespoon Flax Seeds:
Fiber.............3 g
Protein............2g
EPA & DHA.......0
ALA............... 2300 mg
Omega-6..........600 mg
Price......... ....$ .05

Hemp may look like the sore loser, but it's not. Hemp is a pretty well-balanced source of both omega-3 and omega-6. It contains a fairly good ratio of one omega-3 for every three omega-6. If you already get way too much omega-6 in your diet, you may want to go with chia or flax. But consider that hemp is high in protein and chlorophyll. If you look at the color of hemp oil, it is a shade of green. Chlorophyll itself is simply amazing. It is an antioxidant that can bind and remove heavy metals like mercury. Chlorophyll also contains magnesium and can help improve digestion.

Chia is a super-food, hitting all the sweet spots with women. These little black seeds are taken from the plant, Salvia Hispanica. It's got fiber, ALA, it's loaded with minerals, and it's low in omega-6. It does not have an estrogenic effect like flax, and it can be made into a really cool drink. People pay big money for chia drinks in the health food store, but you can easily make your own every day. Just take one tablespoon chia, mix it into some juice and water, and stash it in the fridge, covered. Drink it 1-24 hours later, after it's gelatinous.

Flax is cheap and easy to find, but has pros and cons. The lignans in flax are known to be phytoestrogenic. You should conduct your own research and run it by your doctor to see if they are right for you. If you do choose to supplement with flax, be sure to grind your flax, or get a refrigerated oil, as flax can only be nutritious in this form. Whole flax seeds are useless because your body does not absorb any nutrients from them. Grind them.

You'll notice that none of the seeds contain EPA or DHA. That's why you need algae, fish, or krill oil pills.

How Much is Too Much?

There is no known danger in loading up on omega-3 oils, as long as you still consume some omega-6 oils. Just remember that the more omega-6 you take in, the more your body is going to struggle to make DHA. So pay close attention to the ratio of omega-6 to omega-3. For every one serving of omega-6, be sure to match it with one serving of omega-3.

Although there is no danger of consuming too much omega-3, there is a danger of eating too much fish, as you could develop mercury poisoning and/or PCB toxic overload. If you eat fish, eat it 2-3 times per week, and then supplement with fresh fish oil. Fish oil and algae supplements are made in the lab, where mercury is removed. It makes sense that not all fish oils are created equal. Some are cheap and fishy, others are finer and fresher. Buy a high-quality fish oil to minimize toxins. All algae oil is high-quality because it has not been exploited like the fish oil industry has. The algae oil pills may be expensive, but then you can buy less of the other seed oils and vitamins. You can get more bang for your buck by choosing straight oil over gel caps in both algae and fish oil.

Krill is King

If you want even more bang for your buck, choose krill oil. Krill oil, also known as the king of carotenoids, has several benefits over fish oil. Krill has 20 times more astaxanthin than regular fish oil. Astaxanthin is a red antioxidant which can embed itself in the cell membrane, protecting the cell from ugly free radicals. It is more easily digestible than fish oil. If you are getting the fish burp, it is because of one of two reasons: A. Your bile is not working properly to break down fats like it's

99

supposed to, or B. The oil is too fishy and not fresh enough. Either way, krill oil can help.

Normally after you eat, the liver makes bile and the gallbladder stores the bile. The bile breaks up fat into smaller globules. Then the pancreas does its part by releasing pancreatic lipase, which prepares fat to be further broken down in the small intestine, through emulsification. It is a system. But the system has been broken in many people, and that is why many of us have digestive issues. If your liver is not producing enough bile to break up fat, then you will have a problem digesting fish oil. Krill oil can help. The phospholipid form bypasses the need for emulsification or bile. For anyone who lacks a gallbladder, or has a poorly-functioning gallbladder, this is a close-to-perfect solution. Krill oil is more bioavailable, is more easily absorbed, and bypasses the need for bile and emulsification. And then it has astaxanthin to boot.

In a 2004 comparison study between krill oil and fish oil[31], researchers split 120 participants randomly into four groups. Group A received 2-3 grams krill oil daily; group B received 1-1.5 grams krill oil daily; group C received 3 grams fish oil containing 180mg of DHA and 120mg of EPA three times daily; group D received only a placebo of microcrystalline cellulose. They found that a krill oil supplementation of 1-3 grams (both A and B groups) did the best in terms of managing hyperlipidemia, and reducing glucose (blood sugar), triglycerides (fat), and LDL (bad cholesterol) levels.

Krill oil was even proved effective against arthritis, within 7-14 days of beginning treatment. In 2007, scientists tested its effectiveness on ninety patients who were ill with osteo-arthritis[32], rheumatoid arthritis, or cardiovascular disease. They then tested the patients after 7, 14, and 30 days. After only 7 days, the patients showed that the oil inhibited inflammation and arthritic symptoms at a dose of only 300 mg daily. Amazing!

When you buy your omega-3 supplemental oils, try to buy them from a refrigerator. A good health food store will have a few refrigerated sections not just for food, but for oils and probiotics too. If you cannot find a decent refrigerated source, buy from a trusted online source who likely refrigerates until shipping time. Then you know your oil only spent a few days unrefrigerated, as opposed to it sitting on the grocery store shelf for months. Some online health food retailers even go as far as to ship oils in freezer bags with dry ice. Awesomeness. Also consider purchasing highly perishable oils in the non-summer months if you live in a hot climate. The main oils to be concerned about refrigeration are flax and algae/krill. You may also want to refrigerate hemp as well, though it is not as perishable as flax. You want oils to be perishable, but fresh. Flax oil is least perishable in its seed form. So blending them into your green smoothie is an excellent way to lessen the rancidity.

Oil Pulling

One of my all-time favorite ways to get oils into my system is through oil pulling. Oil pulling is a way to anoint the entire body with oil. The more I oil pull, the better I breathe, the better I look, and the better I feel. When I stop oil pulling, my body becomes overridden with mucous, and I gain weight.

Here is a Basic "how-to":

1. Pour or scoop one tablespoon of coconut oil or sesame oil and place it into your mouth

2. Swish the oil for 15-20 minutes. Do not swallow.
3. Spit the oil into the toilet (or the trash if you are using coconut oil). Cough up as much of the accompanying mucous as you can.
4. Rinse your mouth and brush your teeth.
5. Drink a glass of water.
6. Repeat every morning upon waking. Your stomach should be empty and you should not have anything to drink one hour prior.

Oil pulling has been a complete life-saver for me and for others. It is not a miracle solution, but it will probably bring you where you are going a lot quicker. And it's great for your teeth. If you want to read more about oil pulling, check out "Oil Pulling (The Beauty Books, Volume 1)". It's a must-read if you want to start an effective oil pulling program. If anything, you'll be entertained by my personal story-gone-public.

Chapter Summary

1. Omega 3 oils are fish oil, krill oil, and algae oil. These can be taken in addition to, or instead of eating fish like salmon. Salmon is good, but you can only eat it 2-3 times per week.

2. Omega 6 oils are vegetable oil, soybean oil, canola oil, and corn oil. Limit these as much as you can.

3. Look at your fish oil pill. The amount of any omega-6 vegetable oil you consume should match

the fish oil pill. Eat coconut oil and seed oils liberally; they contain little omega-6.

4. Algae is a much better vegan omega-3 than flax, hemp, and chia because it is bio-available.

Chapter Five

Good Oils, Bad Oils

There are very few oils that are evil. But GMO soybean oil comes to mind. In this chapter, we'll take a look at some of the myths about good oils, and expose some of the bad ones.

Cholesterol

Just because an oil has cholesterol in it, doesn't mean you have a heart disease problem on your hands.

The theory that saturated fat causes heart disease became popular in the 1950's after a researcher checked the diets of inhabitants of seven countries. He found that replacing butter, coconut oil, and lard with polyunsaturated oils like soybean, would lower cholesterol. The researcher, Ancel Keys, then assumed that lowering cholesterol from replacing saturated fats with polyunsaturated fats automatically led to a lower heart disease risk.

However, heart disease has risen to be the number one killer in America. Butter and lard usage has declined dramatically. If we are all eating unsaturated vegetable oil now, shouldn't heart disease decline?

Some experts still say saturated fat causes heart disease, but that doesn't explain how large groups of people can get away with it. The Inuits up in Greenland for instance, eat a diet of mostly fatty meat and fatty seafood, but they don't have a cardiovascular issue. Heart disease is extremely rare there.

And what about Pacific Islanders, eating coconut fat as their main source of fat? 30% of their diet comes from coconut oil. Heart disease is extremely low in these areas. Why aren't they plagued with cardiovascular disease like us?

It simply makes no sense. The theory has too many holes.

I have personally seen my own cholesterol count improve since beginning to use coconut oil. However, I don't attribute this to coconut-eating alone, but to healthier eating in general, taking clever supplements, and working out too. Coconut is my main go-to oil for cooking, as it holds up best under heat. It's the medium-chain fatty acids that make coconut unique and helpful in lowering cholesterol and cutting belly fat.

In a 2009 obesity study[21] which divided women into two groups—Group S who supplemented with soybean oil, and group C who supplemented with coconut oil, researchers found favorable results pointing to coconut oil's ability to improve cholesterol levels and trim fat.

The women in Group C were given about 30 ml (roughly 2 tablespoons) of coconut oil daily. They practiced a healthy diet and a walking routine of 50 minutes per day. The soybean group did the same: 30 ml soybean oil, well-balanced diet, 50 minutes walking. After only a week, the study reported smaller waist circumferences in the women that ate coconut oil.

Group C women had:
Increased levels of HDL (good cholesterol)
Decreased LDL/HDL ratio
Reduced abdominal fat

Group S women had:
Increased total cholesterol
Increased LDL (bad cholesterol)
Increased LDL/HDL ratio
Decreased HDL (good cholesterol)

No reduced abdominal fat

I don't know about you, but I would have begged to be in the coconut group. Who wants to consume tablespoons of soybean oil? Eww. The only "good" thing that happened in that group was that they didn't gain weight.

A similar study exists where scientists compare extra-virgin olive oil and extra-virgin coconut oil. Olive oil was the clear winner. Aha!—you say.

No. No aha. Comparing extra-virgin olive oil to extra-virgin coconut oil is like comparing apples to bananas. You should just eat both. It is silly to compare olive oil to coconut oil because they are two different oils, with two different purposes. Someone needs to hand the researchers this list:

Do not cook with extra-virgin olive oil.
Cook with extra-virgin coconut oil.
Do not make salads with extra-virgin coconut oil.
Make salads with extra-virgin olive oil.

Because you use the oils for separate purposes, there is no need to compare them. Both oils are winners. Consume both. When you cook, use coconut. When you go raw, use olive. Hemp oil works great with raw foods as well.

Many researchers are changing thought about what causes heart disease. We used to believe that saturated fat was the bad guy, but more and more studies are coming forth with evidence that a major contributor to heart disease is arterial plaque, caused by free radical damage.

When a cook pours a polyunsaturated oil on to the pan and heats it up, the oil begins to transform. They are preparing a lovely trans-fat right there in their own kitchen—all for you.

You thank the cook and you eat the yum stuff. Free radicals begin to form inside your body. They damage your cell membranes. They build arterial plaque within your blood vessels. Lastly, you become burdened with other health problems besides cardiovascular disease.

Ok, it's a little far-fetched to say that the damage happens after one meal, but you probably have already heard about the awful effects of trans-fats on the human body. Continued use of trans-fats will likely cause serious health problems. And it will probably make you fatter than you'd like to be too.

What causes heart disease? Could be sugar, processed food-like items, and/or unhealthy oils.

In an article posted at The Weston Price Foundation, Dr. Mary G. Anig and Sally Fallon assert that "triglycerides don't come from dietary fat, but come from excess sugar that have not been used for energy."

Healthy fat just does not translate into belly fat. The Weston Price Foundation is a great resource for finding out about healthy ways of eating. They also run the Real Milk[32] site, which helps you find raw milk and butter in your area.

Pass the Butter

Poor butter. First it was liked, then it was shunned and replaced with processed manufactured spread. Butter is making a small comeback, thanks to Paleo dieters, but is still losing out to its counterpart, margarine.

Is it as evil as people seem to think? Let's examine some facts.

What Vitamins and Minerals Does Butter Have?

- ✓ Vitamin A
- ✓ Vitamin K2
- ✓ Vitamin E
- ✓ Vitamin D
- ✓ Manganese
- ✓ Chromium
- ✓ Zinc
- ✓ Copper
- ✓ Selenium
- ✓ Iodine
- ✓ Essential Fatty Acids—Omega-3 & Omega-6

What Does Butter Do in Your Body?

1. **Supplies Energy:** Butter helps to supply the vital organs with energy.

2. **Combats Heart Disease:** It contains vitamins that protect against heart disease. It has anti-tumor and anti-cancer properties.

3. **Anti-Cancer:** It is particularly the fatty acid, conjugated linoleic acid (CLA), which protects against cancer.

4. **Fights Arthritis:** Butter's got the Wulzen Factor. The Wulzen Factor, discovered by Dutch researcher Rosalind Wulzen, is an anti-stiffness compound that helps with arthritis. It is only found in raw butter and ghee.

5. **Helps Thyroid Gland:** Butter is a rich source of iodine that will help the thyroid gland function

properly. Then, the Glycospingolipids in butter help protect against gastrointestinal infection.

6. **Fights Fatness:** Butter's conjugated linoleic acid and other fatty acids help control weight.

In 2007, researchers reviewed 18 scientific research studies[33] and found that conjugated linoleic acid (CLA) showed a modest reduction in fat mass in obese people, when given at a daily dose of 3.2 grams per day.

However, there is some concern with CLA supplementation. Some studies have shown that it can lead to fatty liver[34], and cause the dreaded insulin resistance[35]. So don't run out and get yourself a whole bottle of the CLA. Just take it in slowly within your grass-fed butter, beef, and milk.

Does butter still sound bad to you? We've all been duped! But before you run out to sink your teeth into some butter, try to find raw butter. Raw butter from grass-fed cows is your best option to get the benefits of butter.

If you cannot find raw, look for grass-fed. The Danish are excellent dairy farmers. Their cows are mostly grass-fed, but they do not make a big deal out of it. They do not talk about it because that's the way it's been for hundreds of years—nothing new and exciting like it is in America. It says nowhere on the packaging, but it just is. A good grass-fed Danish butter brand that you can find in the U.S. is called, "Lurpak," made by Arla.

But remember, it is butter. You still don't want to load up on it, or you'll end up pimply and fat. It's only for times when you need something fattening to spread on your bread besides coconut oil. Reach for real butter instead of the manufactured lab spread, otherwise known as margarine.

I personally can't handle too much butter. One time I ran out of coconut oil. I'm pretty frugal, but I care enormously about my health. I prefer to purchase my coconut oil online from a trusted source, so I can get a good price. Well...I forgot to order one time and ran out for about a week. I swung by the local market and picked up some pastured butter. I decided I would cook everything in grass-fed butter. Smart. Who needs coconut oil when you've got healthy grass-fed butter around the corner?

I put it in and on everything. It changed my whole face. I broke out, looked bloated and felt like a disgusting blob. I know a lot of people swear by pastured butter, and it may be fine and dandy for them, but it's just not my first go-to beauty food. Sorry butter fans. Now I've got it down to just an occasional treat.

Butter from pastured cows does contain more omega-3 than regular butter, but it is such a small amount. If you are trying to get your omega-3 and other vitamins from butter, stop it. Stop trying to get your omega-3 from butter. Its waaay too little omega-3 to get enough. You need 2000-3000 mg of omega-3 per day to lose fat. A full tablespoon of pastured butter won't even give you 100 mg. Pastured butter is a fantastic alternative to eating processed spread, but don't overdo it.

Animal Fats

Animal fats have been used by humans to cook with for hundreds of years. The fat from pig (lard), the fat from cow and mutton (tallow) and the fat from goose have been used long before the manufacture of vegetable oils. Lard used to be the primary source of cooking oil in America before Crisco came in with an all-vegetable shortening high in omega-6 fats. People accepted it as healthier.

Lard contains about 40% saturated fat, 48% monounsaturated fat and 12% polyunsaturated fat. The omega-3 content of lard will depend on what the pig ate. Grass-fed pigs will be higher than that of organic and factory-farmed pigs. Grass-fed pigs are generally hard to find. Though rare, it is not unheard of for a farmer to raise pigs as "pastured," which means they eat natural foods such as bugs, corn, vegetables, fruit, weeds, and some grass. An example of a farm raising pastured pigs, with no commercial feed is the Sugar Mountain Farm in Vermont[36].

It is becoming more common to find pigs raised on organic feed, which means you are getting organic, non-GMO corn, soy, and maybe some grain. Getting organic lard means that you are at least not getting a dose of antibiotics and hormones, but that the omega-6 content is probably still high. There's not much point in trying to consume either pastured or organic lard in hopes of getting EPA and DHA. However, wild boar from the tropics can contain lauric acid and ALA if the pig consumed coconut. But before you write lard completely off, there is one major benefit of lard from pastured pigs: the vitamin D content of a single tablespoon is a whopping 1000 iu's.

Grass-fed beef tallow is a slightly better option than lard when it comes to getting the omega-3. It's not salmon though. Salmon is nearly an overkill when it comes to DHA and EPA, but you can't eat salmon every day. You probably don't want to eat grass-fed beef everyday either, but grass-fed beef will fit in well to your meal rotation. A major benefit of cooking with beef tallow is that your oil is not carcinogenic, like the polyunsaturated vegetable oils.

Like butter, both tallow and lard have their beneficial qualities, but you still don't want to go crazy with them.

Lard is making such a huge comeback, that I'm nearly scared to say this: I do not and will not be eating it. It's not appetizing enough and I find pork fairly disgusting in general. But I do understand and appreciate people choosing it over questionable lab-produced, GMO soybean oil. I personally will not be running to include lard in my list of beauty oils. But if you can pull it off, then have at it.

Grass-fed beef and pork are for people who really enjoy meat and can't live without it. It's futile to force yourself to eat grass-fed animals, if you don't care much for heavy meats. They are more expensive than pastured chicken, they have much less omega-3 than fish, and raising pigs and cattle is unsustainable for our planet.

According to the EPA (Environmental Protection Agency)[37], it takes a staggering 1799 gallons of clean water to make a single pound of beef. Others report that number to be much higher. David Pimentel, in an article entitled "Environmental Sustainability and Integrity in the Agriculture Sector," reported that 12,001 gallons of water was needed to make a pound of beef.

Indeed, raising pastured animals is much better for our planet than conventional animals. But the water waste is there, nonetheless. You are probably wondering about chicken. Oh, it's only 468 gallons to make a pound. And a pound of pork takes 576 gallons. Yeah, it's a lot of water, and a life is being taken, so make sure you really want that grass-fed pound of meat. If you are indifferent about meat, go for the pastured chicken, which takes less water to drink, less water to clean the farmyard, and less water to grow its food. Or better yet go for eggs, and the almighty egg yolk.

Pastured eggs tend to contain about twice as much omega-3 as grain-fed eggs, according to Mother Earth News[38]. When you choose pastured, choose from farms who actually pasture them. Too many farmers just let them roam around in a barn eating corn. Free-range does not necessarily mean pastured.

Indeed, a chicken that is able to roam freely in a barn is always better than a stressed out, cooped up chicken in a cage. A chicken who roams freely in a barn is usually being fed corn and soy or organic corn and organic soy. You don't need either. Your best bet is eggs from a pastured chicken, who roams freely outside eating bugs, worms, fruit, compost, greens, and anything else growing freely. Pastured eggs also contain 7 times more beta-carotene and 3 times more vitamin E.

Vegetable Oils and Margarine

Vegetable oils look and sound pretty, but that's where the beauty ends. Consume these, and you're asking for trouble. The most common perpetrators are soybean oil, canola oil, sunflower oil, corn oil, and safflower oil. Introduced to America as healthier, slimming oils, these oils may just do the opposite. The majority of these oils are not extracted using an expeller-press method. Instead, the oil is chemically removed from the plant, which involves heating to the point where the oil is genetically altered.

Here is a step-by-step glimpse into the making of the oh-so-healthy canola oil[39]:

1. Canola begins as a pretty, genetically-modified yellow summer flower. Farmers harvest seeds from pods which form after flowers die.

2. Machine sieves seeds. Foreign material is collected and sold to farmers as cattle feed.

3. Seeds pass by magnet to remove any metal.

4. Seeds are crushed to thin flakes.

5. Screw-press squeezes flakes with high pressure to force out oil. The brown substance left over after pressing is called, "canola cake." Want some?

6. Canola cake is sent for extraction number two. The second extraction is a 70-minute solvent chemical wash that removes nearly every last trace of oil.

7. Canola cake is grinded and sold as animal feed.

8. Extracted oil is stored in large tanks to await the next stage, the refining phase.

9. Oil is washed for 20 minutes with Sodium Hydroxide, also known as lye.

10. Oil is spun at high speeds to separate "impurities."

11. Impurities are sold to soap manufacturers.

12. Oil is cloudy. Oil is chilled to 41 degrees Fahrenheit to thicken wax and filter.

13. Wax makes vegetable shortening.

14. Oil is bleached to whiten the color.

15. Oil is heat processed with steam injection to remove odor.

16. The "oil" is now refined and ready to bottle.

I'm not sure who has it worse—the animals eating brown canola cake, or us eating lyed and bleached oil-like product. Canola cake—yum!

Seriously though, canola can cause liver damage and cancer. It also can cause imbalance to your brain chemistry, causing violent behavior and the release of stress hormones. Do not try this polyunsaturated oil at home.

It's the over consumption of polyunsaturated oils that doesn't work well within your body. The fat content of the human body is about 97% saturated and monounsaturated fat. Saturated fat is oils like coconut oil, butter, and lard. Monounsaturated fat is oils like olive oil and avocado oil.

Only 3% of our fat composition is polyunsaturated fat. Polyunsaturated fat is the omegas—omega-6 and omega-3 oils. The 3% polyunsaturated in the body is--or should be--about half omega-6 and half omega-3. So what happens when we take in tons of omega-6 and barely any omega-3? Kaboom!

We needed equal parts omega-6 and omega-3. While the standard American diet omega-6 to omega-3 ratio is anywhere from 10:1 to 20:1, it should be more like 1:1, so that the intake can be more like what the human body consists of. Any variation of that will leave you unbalanced and possibly ill.

If the cells are fed lots of omega-6, then the cells will be comprised of omega-6. Omega-6 is an inflammatory fatty acid, so you end up with inflamed cells. If you have inflamed cells, you have an inflamed body. And then you have that bloated appearance, because your entire body is swollen—especially your abdominal area—the area covering your organs. When your organ cells become fatty and inflamed, you feel fat, and it's just not healthy. Water isn't the only way to slim down the belly—omega-3 does it too!

Common polyunsaturated fats include canola oil, sunflower oil, safflower oil, corn oil, and soybean oil. They are also commonly known as just "vegetable oils." These are the oils that most of America has been talked into to using for cooking. Some people are even using them in salads.

Along with the over-consumption, the oils themselves are pretty disturbing. After being heated, lyed, and bleached to have the perfect clear color, it's no wonder that consumers of these chemical oils have illnesses ranging from arthritis to cancer. Who can hold up after 30 years of that abuse?

The factory heating alone causes alteration of the composition. When you consume these oils, you create free radicals inside your body that make you look and feel older. They probably make you look and feel fat too. Your cell membranes begin to be comprised of these damaged oils. A good way to combat the damage is by eating lots of fruits and veggies, which contain antioxidants. Bringing on the veggies, and loading up on omega-3 will slow the effect, and eventually reverse the trend altogether.

Margarine is another factory phenomenon. Margarine is the most horrid version of vegetable oil. It is trans-fat vegetable oil, with a messed-up "healthy" label on the front, confusing everyone who looks at it too long. Just walk on by this factory contraption. Margarine is a fabricated version of butter that was invented around the time that corn and soybean oil came on to the scene in the seventies. They touted that it was healthier than saturated fat. They told us we should not be eating foods that had been eaten for centuries, like butter, lard, and coconut oil. America then proceeded to eat it, and heart disease in America skyrocketed.

If you consume processed food, you will most likely be consuming omega-6 vegetable oils. Read the labels. When you limit processed food, you limit the bad oils, along with a ton of other garbage you don't need. But that's another book. For now, let's just study the oils. Take the good ones in and be beautiful, or consume the bad ones and be ill or unattractive. Processed food includes restaurant food, where you have no idea what the ingredients actually are...let alone what kind of oil and oil temperature that's being used.

I may have a tad social anxiety, but I am a little hesitant to go to a restaurant and dictate what type of ingredients they can or cannot use. This is why I barely eat out, and when I do, I just let it go. You can't win all the time. But if you eat mostly at home, you can better control the ingredients that you put in your mouth. Don't be too busy to provide a nourishing meal for yourself. Your health and your beauty are two of your most important assets. Slow cook your meals in a slow cooker, so it is ready when you get off work. Eat raw meals sometimes that save time on cooking. Or try preparing 3-4 meals on one day.

I've seen many thin & healthy chicks doing this, and I'm jealous. It looks like so much fun.

But just for kicks and giggles, Monsanto is coming out with a genetically modified soybean that is enriched with omega-3[40]. So if you ever see an omega-3 soybean oil sitting on the shelf in the market, run for the hills! The new GMO omega-3 vegetable oil has already been approved by the FDA.

GMO's, or genetically modified organisms already account for a large majority of vegetable oils. Some say about 90% of all canola oil is GMO product, about 93% of all soybeans are genetically modified, and 88% of all corn is genetically modified. So if you have any processed products sitting in your pantry that contain soy, corn, or canola (also known as rapeseed), you are most likely consuming GMO's.

Soybeans are not just genetically modified. They are genetically modified to be Round Up-ready, which means they are able to survive a heavy dousing of pesticide. So you are getting GMO with an extra special pesticide bonus. The main perpetrator in Round Up is glyphosate.

In an Argentinian study published in 2010[41], doctors released the results of the effect of glyphosate when tested on frog and chicken embryos. They found neural and eye defects, undeveloped kidneys and craniofacial malformations. I know we're not frogs, but I'm not waiting to find out the effect on humans. The doctor that headed the study, Andres Carrasco, warned about the risks to unborn babies. He details that abnormally high rates of cancer, kidney, skin, and respiratory diseases are prevalent in residential areas that are nearby soybean farms in Argentina.

Russia even banned GMO's after performing multiple studies[42] showing the detrimental effect of the genetically modified soybean on the reproductive systems of animals. The

Russians caught on very quickly. They got it. Why can't we? What's the hold up in the U.S.?

Chapter Summary

1. Processed omega-6 oils can be detrimental to health. Limit these.

2. Recent studies have shown that saturated fat does not cause heart disease.

3. Eat pastured meat and dairy. It contains less omega-6 and more omega-3.

Last Thoughts

If you take one thing from this book with you, know that you need good fat to get rid of bad fat. Good fats will nourish your cells so that they can do their work. Good fats, like castor oil will stimulate fat and get it moving. You want to stimulate fat, because it will be easier to move out of the body when the cells liven and begin to work.

Stagnation=Belly Fat

One of the best ways to increase movement is to get moving. You already know how important exercise is to looking healthy, young, and beautiful. Keep on working out. Don't ever stop. Your knowledge of how oils work is just an extra advantage point now.

Many people that workout struggle with belly fat. The older you get, the more belly you've got. It's totally normal to be working out and doing the best you can, but still have trouble losing the gut. That's because abs are made in the kitchen. No amount of sit-ups are going to trim the belly if you've got poundage of fat on it. Sure, you can build the abdominal muscles underneath, but you still look pot-bellyish because the fat is still there on top. You probably can't see your six pack because it is hiding under all the fat. That's the way it works with the belly. You can have muscles and fat hanging off at the same time. In order to see the muscles, you have to trim the fat first. Work the main muscle groups in the gym: legs, back, chest. Do some abs—sure--but then use the principles in this book, to trim the last bit of fat.

If you have never cleansed before, try a parasite cleanse first. Then move on to specific areas you would like to work on—the Olive Oil Cleanse mentioned in this book is an excellent way to clear up the liver and gallbladder so that they can function better. That's what cleanses are all about. You want to clear away as much junk as possible so that your organs can do what they need to do. If you have trouble digesting and processing fat, give your liver some space. Clear away toxins. It takes an enormous amount of energy to digest food. Your liver can use a hand sometimes. Try not to overburden it with binge drinking, overeating, and pills. The market is flooded with colon cleanses. Cleansing the colon is extremely important, but the colon is not all there is. We have our liver, gallbladder, lungs, kidneys, and ovaries to keep clean and functioning as well.

If you already eat fairly clean, and have been doing different organ cleanses for a while, use the castor oil packs for several days once a month. Do not use the packs while on your period—just let your body do its thing. Periods are a way for your body to cleanse, so be grateful! It's a free cleanse and your subscription is automatically renewed every month. If your periods are irregular, still be grateful, but try to get on the regular train as soon as you can. Get hormone tests done at the doctor's office. Use the castor oil packs liberally, and also try Chinese herbal tampons to clear any toxins and blockage.

Remember, there is no miracle solution. Your health and beauty are two of your greatest assets. Don't neglect them or cover up with synthetic materials. Sure, it's fun to put on a little make-up and dress up. But every now and then, dedicate some time to figuring out how to wake up beautiful. Good oils will help you glow and thrive naturally.

One Last Thing Before You Go

Thank you sooo much for purchasing this book and reading it. I hope you have enjoyed reading it as much as I have enjoyed writing it. I would be honored and grateful if you posted a review of this book here on Amazon and/or share your thoughts of this book with your friends. It will help other readers find the book. They want flat bellies too!

Sources

1. Smith, Gall, McNaugton, Blizzard, Dwyer, and AJ Venn. "Skipping breakfast: longitudinal associations with cardiometabolic risk factors in the Childhood Determinants of Adult Health Study." The American Journal of Clinical Nutrition. December 2010.

2. Shapiro, Tumer, Gao, Cheng, and PJ Scarpace. "Prevention and reversal of diet-induced leptin resistance with a sugar-free diet despite high fat content." The British Journal of Nutrition. August 2011.

3. Thorburn, Stolien, Jenkins, Khouri, and EW Kraegen. "Fructose-induced in vivo insulin resistance and elevated plasma triglyceride levels in rats." The American Journal of Clinical Nutrition. 1989.

4. St-Onge, and Jones PJ. "Greater rise in fat oxidation with medium-chain triglyceride consumption relative to long-chain triglyceride is associated with lower initial body weight and greater loss of subcutaneous adipose tissue." International Journal of Obesity and Related Metabolic Disorders. December 2003.

5. St-Onge, Borque, Jones, Ross, and WE Parsons. "Medium- versus long-chain triglycerides for 27 days increases fat oxidation and energy expenditure without resulting in changes in body composition in overweight women."

International Journal of Obesity and Related Metabolic Disorders. January 2003.

6. Loenneke, Wilson, Manninen, Wray, Barnes, and T Pujol. "Quality protein intake is inversely related with abdominal fat." Nutrition and Metabolism. Jan 2012.

7. Leidy, Ortinau, Rains, and Kevin Maki. "Acute effects of higher protein, sausage and egg-based convenience breakfast meals on postprandial glucose homeostasis in healthy, premenopausal women (381.6)." The Journal of the Federation of American Societies for Experimental Biology. April 2014.

8. Leidy, Ortinau, Douglas, and Heather A Hoertel. "Beneficial effects of a higher-protein breakfast on the appetitive, hormonal, and neural signals controlling energy intake regulation in overweight/obese, "breakfast-skipping," late-adolescent girls." The American Journal of Clinical Nutrition. February 2013.

9. Lee, John R. John Lee MD, Your Information Source for Hormone Balance and Natural HRT. Web. n.d.

10. The Weston A. Price Foundation. The Weston A. Price Foundation for Wise Traditions in Food, Farming, and the Healing Arts. Web. n.d.

11. Frazier, Matt. No Meat Athlete. Web. n.d.

12. "Uterine Fibroids Symptoms, Diagnosis, and Treatment." Society of Interventional Radiology. Web. n.d.

13. "Uterine Fibroid Facts Sheet." Womenshealth.gov. Office on Women's Health, U.S. Department of Health and Human Services. Web. n.d.

14. McGarey, William A. The Oil that Heals: A Physician's Successes with Castor Oil Treatments. Virginia Beach: A.R.E. Press, 2002. Print.

15. Grady Harvey. "Immunomodulation through castor oil packs." Journal of Naturopathic Medicine. 1999; 7(1):84-8916.

16. "Final Report on the Safety Assessment of Ricinus Communis (Castor) Seed Oil, Hydrogenated Castor Oil, Glyceryl Ricinoleate, Glyceryl Ricinoleate SE, Ricinoleic Acid, Potassium Ricinoleate, Sodium Ricinoleate, Zinc Ricinoleate, Cetyl Ricinoleate, Ethyl Ricinoleate, Glycol Ricinoleate, Isopropyl Ricinoleate, Methyl Ricinoleate, and Octyldodecyl Ricinoleate." International Journal of Toxicology. May 2007.

17. Medhi, Kishore, Singh, and SD Seth. "Castor Oil is Safe and Effective in the treatment of patients with osteoarthritis." Phytother Res. October 2009.

18. Vieira, Fetzer, Sauer, Evangelista, Averbeck, Kress, Reeh, Cirillo, Lippi, Maggi, and S Manzini. "Pro- and anti-inflammatory actions of ricinoleic acid: similarities and differences with capsaicin." Naunyn-Schmiedeberg Arch Pharmacol. 2001 Aug;364(2):87-95.

19. "Slideshow: A Visual Guide to Uterine Fibroids." Web MD. Web. April 2014.

20. Seaton, Welle, Warenko, and RG Campbell. "Thermic effect of medium-chain and long-chain triglycerides in man." The American Journal of Clinical Nutrition. 1986.

21. Asuncao, Ferreira, dos Santos, Cabral, and TM Florencio. "Effects of dietary coconut oil on the biochemical and anthropometric profiles of women presenting abdominal obesity." Lipids. 2009 Jul;44(7):593-601.

22. Fife, Bruce. Coconut Oil Miracle. New York: Penguin, 2004. Print.

23. Oi-Kano, Kawada, Watanabe, Koyama, Watanabe, Senbongi, and K Iwai. "Oleuropein, a phenolic compound in extra virgin olive oil, increases uncoupling protein 1 content in brown adipose tissue and enhances noradrenaline and adrenaline secretions in rats." Journal of Nutritional Science and Vitaminology. 2008 Oct;54(5):363-70.

24. Technische Universitaet Muenchen. "Olive oil makes you feel full." ScienceDaily. 14 March 2013.

25. Clark, Hulda. "Liver Cleanse, Gallbladder Cleanse, Liver Flush." Cure Zone. Web. 1995.

26. Sabate, Joan. "Nut consumption and body weight." The American Journal of Clinical Nutrition. 2003.

27. Rastrollo, Wedick, Martinez-Gonzalez, Li, Sampson, and Frank Hu. The American Journal of Clinical Nutrition. 2009.

28. Smith, Atherton, Reeds, Mohammed, Rankin, Rennie, and Bettina Mittendorfer. "Dietary omega-3 fatty acid supplementation increases the rate of muscle protein synthesis in older   adults: a randomized controlled trial." American Journal of Clinical Nutrition. 2011.

29. Jenkins, Mark. "Antioxidants and Free radicals." Rice University. Web. 1996.

30. Dangardt, Osika, Chen, Nilsson, Gan, Gronowitz, Strandvik, and Friberg. "Omega-3 fatty acid supplementation improves vascular function and reduces inflammation in obese adolescents." Atherosclerosis. 2010 Oct;212(2):580-5.

31. Deutsch, L. "Evaluation of the effect of Neptune Krill Oil on chronic inflammation and arthritic symptoms." Journal of the American College of Nutrition. 2007 Feb;26(1):39-48.

32. "Home: The Facts About Real Raw Milk." Real Milk. The Weston A. Price Foundation. Web. 2015.

33. Whigham, Watras, and Dale Schoeller. "Efficacy of conjugated linoleic acid for reducing fat mass: a meta-analysis in humans." The American Journal of Clinical Nutrition. 2007.

34. Vyas, Kumar, Kadegowda, and Richard Erdman. "Dietary Conjugated Linoleic Acid and Hepatic Steatosis: Species-Specific Effects on Liver and Adipose Lipid Metabolism and Gene   Expression." Journal of Nutrition and Metabolism. 2012.

35. Riserus, Arner, Brismar, and Bengt Vessby. "Treatment With Dietary trans10cis12 Conjugated Linoleic Acid Causes Isomer-Specific Insulin Resistance in Obese Men With the Metabolic Syndrome." American Diabetes Association Diabetes Care. 2002.

36. Jeffries, Walter. "Hay's Here 2011 – Pigs Eat Grass!" Sugar Mountain Farm. Web. 2011.

37. Catanese, Christina. "Virtual Water, Real Impacts: World Water Day 2012." EPA. Web. March 2012.

38. Long, and Tabitha Alterman. "Meet Real Free-Range Eggs." Mother Earth News. Web. 2007.

39. Panos Egglezos. "How It's Made—Canola Oil." Online Video Clip. You Tube. March 11, 2012.

40. "Omega-3-Enhanced Soybean Oil." Monsanto. Web. n.d.

41. Carrasco, Andres. "Teratogenesis by glyphosate based herbicides and other pesticides.
Relationship with the retinoic acid pathway." Molecular Embryology, School of Medicine UBA. 2013.

42. Smith, Jeffrey. "Genetically Modified Soy Linked to Sterility, Infant Mortality in Hamsters." The Huffington Post. Web. August 2010.

43. Hill, Buckley, Murphy, and Peter Howe. "Combining Fish oil Supplements with regular aerobic excersize improves

body composition and cardiovascular disease risk factors." The American Journal of Clinical Nutrition. May 2007.

44. Fulgoni, Dreher, and Adrienne Davenport. "Avocado consumption is associated with better diet quality and nutrient intake, and lower metabolic syndrome risk in US adults: results from the National Health and Nutrition Examination Survey. Nutrition Journal. 2013, 12:1.

Other Sources

"Addendum A: EPA and DHA Content of Fish Species." health.gov. Appendix G2: Original Food Guide Pyramid Patterns and Description of USDA Analyses. n.d.

"All About Fish Eggs." Paleo Leap. Web. June 2014.

Ash, Michael. "The Forgotten Therapeutic Applications of Castor Oil." Clinical Education. Web. 16 April 2013.

Bailey, Regina. "Thymus." About Education. http://biology.about.com/od/anatomy/ss/thymus.htm. n.d.

Besdine, Richard. "Changes in the Body With Aging." Merck Manuals. Web. December 2013.

Bes-Rastrollo, Wedick, Martinez-Gonzalez, Li, Sampson, and Frank Hu. The American Journal of Clinical Nutrition. June 2009 vol. 89 no. 6 1913-1919.

Brain, Marshall. "How Your Immune System Works" 01 April 2000. HowStuffWorks.com. <http://health.howstuffworks.com/human-body/systems/immune/immune-system.htm> 19 March 2015.

Byrnes, Stephen. "Why Butter is Better." Mercola.com. Web. March 31, 2001.

"Convention." Minamata Convention On Mercury. UNEP. Web. n.d.

CTVNews.ca Staff. "U.S. Study looks into the benefits of coconut oil on patients with Alzheimer's." CTV News. October 9, 2013.

Dansinger, Michael. "What is Metabolic Syndrome." Web MD. Web. December 21, 2013.

Drobot, and Dickson Thom. "Castor Oil: An Essential for Health." The American Center for Biological Medicine, The Marion Institute.n.d.

Dyer, and Amy DiCioccio. "Flaxseeds and Breast Cancer." Oncology Nutrition. Academy of Nutrition and Dietetics. January 2014.

Enos, Deborah. "Go Nuts and Still Lose Weight." Live Science. Web. May 8, 2013.

Erasmus, Udo. Fats That Heal, Fats That Kill. Summertown: Alive Books. 1993.

"Extra-Virgin Olive Oil-Thermogenic and Anabolic!" Advanced Muscle Science Lab.Web. August 21 2012.

Fallon, and Mary Enig. "The Skinny on Fats." The Weston A. Price Foundation. Web. January 1, 2000.

"Gallstones." Liver.ca. Canadian Liver Foundation. Web. n.d.

"Health Benefits of Grass-Fed Products." Eat Wild. Web. n.d. Accessed 02/15/2015.

Jacob, Aglaee. "Coconut Oil—Learn More About This Superfood That Contains Healthful Saturated Fats." Today's Dietitian. Vol.15 No.10 P.56. October 2013.

Kelly, Margie. "Top 7 Genetically Modified Crops." The Huffington Post. October 2012.

Koh, Lee WJ, Lee SA, Kim EH, Cho, Jeong, Kim DW, Kim Ms, Park JY, Park KG, Lee HJ, Lee IK, Lim, Jang, Lee KH, and KU Lee. "Effects of alpha-lipoic Acid on body weight in obese subjects." American Journal of Medicine. 2011 Jan;124(1):85.e1-8.

Masterjohn, Christopher. "Fatty Acid Analysis of Grass-fed and Grain-fed Beef Tallow." The Weston A. Price Foundation. Web. January 21, 2014.

Masterjohn, Christopher. "Good Fats, Bad Fats: Separating Fact from Fiction." The Weston A. Price Foundation. Web. January 1, 2012.

Matthews, Michael. "How Much Protein is Needed to Build Muscle." Muscle For Life. Web. n.d.

Messina, Virginia. "The Fatty Acids." Veganhealth.org. Web. n.d.

Munro and Garg Manohar. "Dietary supplementation with long chain omega-3 polyunsaturated fatty acids and weight loss in obese adults." ResearchGate. Obesity Research and Clinical Practice. University of Newcastle. 05/2013; 7(3):e173-e181

Norris, Jack. "Omega-3 Fatty Acid Recommendations for Vegetarians." Veganhealth.org. Web. April 2014.

Nutrition Examination Survey (NHANES) 2001–2008." Nutrition Journal. January 2013.

"Omega-3 Fatty Acids." The World's Healthiest Foods. Web. n.d.

Paganelli, Gnazzo, Acosta, Lopez, and Andres Carrasco. "Glyphosate-Based Herbicides Produce Teratogenic Effects on Vertebrates by Impairing Retinoic Acid Signaling." Chemical Research   in Toxicology. August 2010. 23 (10), pp 1586–1595.

Patrick, and M Uzick. "Cardiovascular disease: C-reactive protein and the inflammatory disease paradigm: HMG-CoA reductase inhibitors, alpha-tocopherol, red yeast rice, and olive oil   polyphenols. A review of the literature." Alternative

Medicine Review: a Journal of Clinical Therapeutic. 2001, 6(3):248-271.

Reinagel, Monica. "Chia vs. Hemp vs. Flax." Quick and Dirty Tips. Web. February 2013.

Self Nutrition Data, Know What You Eat. Conde Nast. Web. n.d. Accessed 02/15/2015.

Sherry, Amelia R. "Spotlight on Stearidonic Acid — Learn More About This Alternative Omega-3 Fatty Acid." Today's Dietitian. July 2014. Vol. 16 No. 7 P. 18.

"Turning up the Heat on Brown Fat." Joslin Diabetes Center. Harvard Medical School. Web. n.d.

Vieira, Evangelista, Cirillo, Lippi, Maggi, and Manzini. "Effect of ricinoleic acid in acute and subchronic experimental models of inflammation." Mediators of Inflammation. 2000; 9(5): 223–   228.

"What do Chickens Eat on Pasture?" The Walden Effect.March 25, 2011.

"What's New and Beneficial About Avocados." The World's Healthiest Foods. Web. n.d.

Wikipedia contributors. "Castor oil." Wikipedia, The Free Encyclopedia. Wikipedia, The Free Encyclopedia. 14 Mar. 2015. Web. 19 Mar. 2015.

Wikipedia contributors. "Ricinoleic acid." Wikipedia, The Free Encyclopedia. Wikipedia, The Free Encyclopedia. 31 Oct. 2014. Web. 19 Mar. 2015.

About the Author

Sonja Larsen is an American living in Denmark with her Danish hubby. She loves devouring healthy things, and has a fondness for oils. She graduated from University of California at Santa Barbara with a B.A. in English Literature and has always loved writing. She is absolutely delighted that the digital age makes it possible for everyone to connect and share. But she does like to power down at the house every once in a while to sip some tea and chillax with an old-fashioned pen and paper.

Sonja loves people. Please contact her at sonjalarsen@outlook.com with questions and/or just to say hi. She'd also be overjoyed if you joined The Beauty Books newsletter at www.thebeautybooks.com.

Other Books by Sonja Y. Larsen:

Oil Pulling (The Beauty Books, Book 1)

www.ingramcontent.com/pod-product-compliance
Lightning Source LLC
Chambersburg PA
CBHW070921290526
45795CB00001B/382